# LOOK TEN YEARS YOUNGER

---

# LIVE TEN YEARS LONGER

## A WOMAN'S GUIDE

### DR. DAVID RYBACK

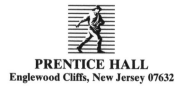

**PRENTICE HALL**
Englewood Cliffs, New Jersey 07632

10   9   8   7   6   5   4   3   2

This book cannot and must not replace hands on medical care or the
specific advice of your doctor. Use it instead to help you ask the right
questions, make the right choices, and work more closely with your
doctor and the other members of your health-care team.

**Library of Congress Cataloging-in-Publication Data**

Ryback, David.
    Look ten years younger, live ten years longer : a woman's guide /
David Ryback.
        p.     cm.
    Includes index.
    ISBN 0–13–079328–0 (cloth)     ISBN 0–13–079310–8 (paper)
    1. Women—Health and hygiene.    2. Longevity.    I. Title.
RA778.R98     1995
613'.04244—dc20
                                                    95–35882
                                                       CIP


ISBN 0-13-079328-0 (C)
ISBN 0-13-079310-8 (P)

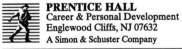
**PRENTICE HALL**
Career & Personal Development
Englewood Cliffs, NJ 07632
A Simon & Schuster Company

On the World Wide Web at http://www.phdirect.com

PRINTED IN THE UNITED STATES OF AMERICA

# CONTENTS

## CHAPTER

# 1

## GROWING OLD, STAYING YOUNG—1

## CHAPTER

# 2

## DR. RYBACK'S ANTIAGING FOOD PLAN—21

**CHAPTER**

**3**

## EXERCISE AWAY THE YEARS—73

**CHAPTER**

# 4

## ANTIAGING STRESS REDUCERS—93

**CHAPTER**

# 5

## MIDLIFE: A RITE OF PASSAGE—123

**CHAPTER**

# 6

# ANTIAGING SEXUALITY AND REPRODUCTIVE HEALTH—151

**CHAPTER**

# 7

# KEEPING YOUR BONES YOUNG—183

**CHAPTER**

# 8

# AGE-PROOFING YOUR SKIN, HAIR, AND TEETH—205

## CHAPTER
# 9

## KEEPING YOUR HEART STRONG AND YOUNG—239

## CHAPTER
# 10

## STOP SMOKING AND ADD YEARS TO YOUR LIFE—267

CHAPTER

# 11

## THINK YOUNG AND BE YOUNG—287

CHAPTER

# 12

## MINIMIZING LIFE PROBLEMS TO LIVE LONGER—309

# FOREWORD

A funny thing happened to me while reading this book—several people commented to me that I looked younger than my years. I could attribute those comments to coincidence, but I prefer to believe that as I absorbed the knowledge in this book and made some small but significant changes in my life (taking vitamins, eating smaller meals, increasing my exercise), I was empowering myself as a woman and starting to present a younger Dr. McCloud. I must admit that I was both proud and pleased to hear the words, "You look younger—what have you been doing differently?"

Now, I would never admit that I want to look ten years younger, but I can publicly proclaim that I want to live ten years longer. And I want those extra ten years to be vital and active. I am assured, as I read this book, and if I follow the simple advice, that I will not only live longer, but that I will feel and be more youthful, as well as lead a more active, productive life. Dr. Ryback grabbed my attention and woke me up to my choices. I am empowered thinking about what I might do to battle the aging process rather than pretending it won't happen to me.

As an obstetrician/gynecologist, I spend my professional life helping my patients become healthier women. I read and learn, ask and probe, prescribe and suggest—all as a matter of course. That's the life of a doctor. With this book, however, I was reminded to focus on myself. I felt as though Dr. Ryback were talking to me directly, about so many of the issues I'd been thinking about as a woman and sharing with other women as patients and friends.

I began Dr. Ryback's book with great interest. As a medical doctor, I know how difficult it is for women to discuss their concerns such as menopause and fear of cancer. Each woman has her own story. To one it might be premature menopause; for another, it might be the sense of appearing disfigured subsequent to fighting breast cancer; to yet another, it might be a pattern of female symptoms that are impossible to diagnose despite months of worry and thousands of dollars of tests.

Most women don't know nearly enough about their bodies and women's health issues. Many are too frightened to find answers to their questions, or even know where to begin. One by one, in simple and concise manner, Dr. Ryback answers the many questions that so many women wonder about. So much information is readily available in this easy-to-read book.

Sex is one topic often ignored in popular books about health. Dr. Ryback has a thoughtful attitude as to what goes into maintaining and improving a healthy sexual relationship. His matter of fact, frank and open manner provides both the knowledge and permission to place sex in the proper perspective. It is as important to a woman's emotional health as are diet and exercise. He encourages women to take charge of their sexuality and enjoy it throughout their adult lives. How wonderfully refreshing!

Reading Dr. Ryback's book was an inspiration to me. In a clear, concise, well-organized fashion, he battles the myth of the "super-woman." According to this myth, not only are we women supposed to be accomplished in our careers, but we're also expected to be nurturing beings, attractive, good-natured, and so on. Dr. Ryback dispels this myth by allowing us to see the destructive forces that emanate from this. He reminds us to take care of ourselves and attend to our stress levels. He appreciates our needs for relationship and offers suggestions to enhance that aspect of our lives.

Dr. Ryback puts the brakes to our crazy, hectic lifestyles. He gives us permission to earn and enjoy those extra ten years. He reminds us of the severe consequences of running tense, trying to squeeze in all those responsibilities as we try to do it all ourselves—family, friends, career. Ahh—the gift of slowing down! Dr. Ryback reframes life's goals so that the real benefits are revealed, while at the same time allowing us to anticipate a longer, fuller life.

Thank you, Dr. Ryback, for writing the book that we women need to read. Thanks for sifting through the hordes of information, integrating and interpreting all of it and then presenting it to us in a way that we can easily utilize to create our best selves. I appreciate the range of topics as well as the message that says: It's up to us, that we can easily make changes and powerful choices that will allow us to live ten years longer and look ten years younger. We have the choices. We can empower ourselves.

**—Melody T. McCloud, M.D. (Ob/Gyn)**
*Author, "Medical Bloopers"*

# INTRODUCTION

## HOW THIS BOOK WILL MAKE YOU
## LOOK YOUNGER AND LIVE LONGER

Sophia Loren, Oscar-winning actress in 1961 for her dramatic role in *Two Women*, is an excellent example of a woman who looks ten years younger than her real age. Turning 60 on September 20, just one year ago, was not traumatic for her, she said, "because I have in my life what I always wanted."

How does she stay so young? By being "a little careful" about her diet and exercising 30 to 40 minutes each day. From her home in Geneva, she shared: "Even I can't believe I'm 60 years old. I feel like I'm 12. I think you have to face reality as it is and you have to go on and find new motivations in your life and new achievements to be able to survive."

"Aging is not 'lost youth' but a new stage of opportunity and strength," writes Betty Friedan, author of *The Feminine Mystique* and, more recently, *The Fountain of Age*. A youthful 74 years of age at the time of this writing, Ms. Friedan sees her mature years as "a new period in life, as yet mostly unknown and untested."

Since 1900, the average lifespan has practically doubled—from 47 to 76. Beyond this statistic, many mature women are finding new challenges and careers as they begin their 60s, 70s, and 80s. One of my patients, Clara, is 80 years old and still swims almost on a daily basis. She even occasionally consults with others from her base of experience as a literary agent. Betty Friedan has a few suggestions for such stalwart women:

1. Cherish your choices and maintain control of your own life.

2. Commit yourself to your passions in work and love.

3. Risk being yourself, who you really are.

4. Risk new things, risk new ways, risk failing.

Never before has there been such a national obsession with longevity. Women among the aging Baby Boomer Generation are courting longer life by focusing on virtually every facet of health and fitness. Nor is this a desire for mere fantasy. Scientists are discovering that people can live much longer than they have been. Census figures reveal and predict a gradually longer average lifespan. According to the Census Bureau, for example, the United States has 36,000 people over the age of 100, and by the year 2020, there will be 266,000.

Two-thirds of Americans want to live 100 years, according to a survey released by the Alliance for Aging Research, a Washington-based research group. Each of us can live to the age of 120, according to UCLA scientist Roy Walford. His theory is based on his own hard data as well as data reported by Clive McKay in 1935. By minimizing calories and providing the correct nutrients, and by developing a healthier lifestyle in general our lives can be extended quite significantly. But very few have done it—yet!

In a recent survey at Northwestern University, which includes a number of studies over a twenty-year period, about 400,000 individuals were analyzed in terms of their lifestyles with regard to health factors. "Clean-living" people—non-smokers with low cholesterol levels—were compared with their high-cholesterol, smoking, high-blood-pressure counterparts. The results? A statistical analysis revealed that those who live a healthier lifestyle actually live 5 to 9 years longer. By purposefully taking control of such health factors as nutrition, fitness, stress reduction, and dealing appropriately with such challenges as menopause and osteoporosis, you can do even better. You can make a proactive choice to look ten years younger and live ten years longer.

For the first time, a comprehensive approach to nutrition, fitness and other aspects of health awareness makes the conservative promise of ten more youthful, healthy years of life real.

Despite a male-dominated medical opinion that research on women's cardiovascular problems is of secondary importance to the study of men, over 500,000 women die of heart disease each year. Yet funds for medical research on women's health issues are hard to come by, relative to those for men. In the field of health care, according to the former Director of the National Institutes of Health (NIH), Bernadine Healy, "women have all too often been treated less than equally."

According to a 1979 study conducted at the University of California at San Diego, men's complaints of back pain, chest pain, dizziness, fatigue and headache more often resulted in extensive work-ups than did similar complaints from women. Though heart disease is the number one killer for both men and women, sophisticated and complex heart operations such as by-pass surgery are prescribed more frequently for men.

Research on diseases unique to women, according to a NIH report, amounted to less than 14 percent of the total research budget. But finally things are beginning to change. In 1991, Representative Patricia Schroeder sponsored legislation to ensure that biomedical research would no longer overlook women and their health. Then the NIH launched the $600 million Women's Health Initiative, a 15-year program to study the effects of estrogen therapy, diet and exercise on heart disease, breast cancer, colon cancer and osteoporosis in 160,000 postmenopausal women.

In 1993, the President stated: "When it comes to health-care research and delivery, women can no longer be treated as second-class citizens." The medical gender gap is finally beginning to close.

Women's health-care concerns—PMS, breast and uterine cancer, osteoporosis, endometriosis, and menopause—are now more clearly recognized as having equal significance to men's health issues. An American Hospital Association survey of over 3,000 hospitals with health-promotion programs found that virtually one-half of these hospitals provided programs especially aimed at women, often in terms of availability of women's health centers.

In cities such as Atlanta, Los Angeles, Portland and a number of others, women can now avail themselves of Feminist Women's Health Centers, where they'll find nonsexist, nonhierarchical medical systems prevailing. In Chicago, the Health Evaluation and Referral Service (HERS) has been providing information to help women transform medical providers to have greater sensitivity to women's health needs since 1973. In these difficult economic times, medical care providers can no longer ignore women, who consume about 60 percent of health-care services in the U.S., as an important sector of the health-care market.

XVIII                                                          INTRODUCTION

This book covers the most important aspects of such nutrition, fitness, and women's lifestyle issues in a simple, yet personal format. It cuts through the morass of overwhelming information and provides a coherent, straightforward series of suggestions targeted for the intelligent woman who is willing to take responsibility for a longer, healthier, happier life.

Look Ten Years Younger, Live Ten Years Longer is an easy read, backed by scientific research, that promises and delivers the information you need to achieve ten more years of youthful life and appearance.

Given the choice of just plain getting older or maturing youthfully, which would you prefer? Looking ten years younger and living ten years longer is definitely within your reach. Do you want to lose weight easily and forever with little effort? Then read about my Antiaging Food Plan and the importance of three-month cycles in losing weight forever. Want to acquire a fitness program that makes you sexier and increases your life span by at least ten percent? Read about my SPEAR approach and enjoy exercising for a more fit, more attractive body. Want smoother, younger skin? Learn the natural path to a youthful look. Give up smoking, when you're ready, by going through a four-step process and using the best quit-smoking technologies available. Learn the brief, simple steps to detect breast, ovarian, uterine and cervical cancers and give up worry for peace of mind. Learn about getting the stress out of your relationships by making better choices and acting wisely so that you can live not only longer but more happily as well. Deal with menopause and osteoporosis effectively so you can enjoy the prime of your life. And as you enjoy ten more years of a youthful life, learn how to "fine-tune" those extra years through specific suggestions for an active and satisfying sex life with your mate through the maturing years.

Never before have women been more aware of nutrition, fitness, and general lifestyle enhancement. Some changes, such as avoiding obesity, quitting smoking, and preventing cancer are obvious. Others, such as learning the optimal dosage of vitamin C (different for each individual), reversing high blood pressure without medication, dealing effectively with menopause and how having reliable support groups affects the aging process, are less obvious. This book explores each of these areas thoroughly, clearing up the confusion that many feel.

All of us wish for extended youth and a longer life. Most of us would be willing to do what it takes to accomplish this if we had simple directions or guidelines that were 1.) scientifically valid, 2.) delivered in a credible style, in 3.) an easily read and understood format.

My main purpose in writing *Look Ten Years Younger, Live Ten Years Longer* was to offer a comprehensive resource that would appeal to those of you who are interested in youth and life extension but have been disappointed by quick-fix remedies and scientifically unsound advice which fail in the end.

You've probably become cynical. You've heard of and tried many diets. You've seen Oprah through her Optifast disaster. You've seen others go down with cancer, despite all attempts at "new age" cures. You're ready for some scientifically sound, simple truth: What really works, why, and how to do it in the most simple, direct way. This book serves that purpose.

The sad truth about longevity is that because some people will not follow through on the healthy lifestyle I recommend in this book, one third of Americans will die of heart disease; over 46,000 women will succumb to breast cancer each year, a form of cancer which could be prevented in part by proper nutrition, good fitness habits, and early detection; over 10,000 women will die of cancer of the cervix and uterus; over 13,000 will die of ovarian cancer.

I am confident that, by following through on my suggestions in this book, backed up by scientific research and consolidated to comprise a simple lifestyle approach, you can confidently take action to help prevent such cancers and anticipate ten more years of healthy life—and looking up to ten years younger than you do now, depending on how different your current lifestyle is from what you read in this book.

Get ready to learn about all of the following:

1. How being more aware of your eating habits and making breast self-exams a routine experience can help you in your own personal campaign against cancer;

2. Guaranteed loss of weight without any strict diet or calorie counting;

3. How the right amount of exercise results in higher sex drive;

4. Scientific evidence that exercising can extend your lifespan significantly;

5. How to cure high blood pressure without medication;

6. How to quit smoking despite the likelihood of initial failures;

7. Coping with stress;

8. A direct approach to sexual problems as you get older.

An intriguing chapter, titled "Midlife: A Rite of Passage," strikes a chord in all women: how to deal with the inevitable aspects of menopause; how to remain youthful despite the advancing years; how to stay sexy and remain lovable.

We all know well the benefits of fitness and good nutrition, and the dangers of obesity and smoking. But this book offers a comprehensive, scientific, yet personal exploration that uncovers the best of what really works and clears up the confusion that surrounds these topics. By following through on the simple suggestions offered in this book, you can confidently look forward to living ten years longer and looking ten years younger.

I've spent the last few years researching the relevant literature and analyzing the lifestyle of my patients as well as my own. I've integrated this with my professional experiences lecturing in the U.S., Europe and Asia, as well as with findings in my own clinical practice.

In this book, I share with you the results of my efforts. You will learn not only how to acquire better eating habits and ways to change values about physical fitness, but also how to enjoy a better love life, and how to make attitudinal and social changes that last. In many little ways, you will learn how to improve the quality of your life that will add up to a significant transformation.

Here is my promise: By opening this book, you've already taken the first step to becoming a healthier, more vital and more youthful woman. If you read, reread and follow through on my suggestions, within a three- to six-month period you will begin to notice a loss in weight, a feeling of greater vitality and an improvement in the romantic and social aspects of your life, both at home and at work.

This is the first time all these factors have been combined in a single book that is based on sound research, yet remains a personalized and comfortable read. *Look Ten Years Younger, Live Ten Years Longer* offers you a combination of personal experience and scientific objectivity, of in-depth, practical advice with a comprehensive range of health topics.

By following through on the recommendations of this book, you can stay healthier, look younger and live longer. How much? Well, that depends on your genetic disposition, the present condition of your body, your degree of commitment, your present age, and where you live. To round it off to the most accurate number to cover the wide divergence among all readers, I feel very comfortable with the number 10. For some women it may be more, for others less. But what's really important is that by following through, you *will* be healthier, with stronger heart and lungs, a smarter, more responsive brain, a more attractive body, and more fulfilling relationships.

# GROWING OLD, STAYING YOUNG

## CHAPTER 1

The potential for extending your life is now greater than ever. Although many have been brainwashed to believe that much of the physical deterioration associated with growing older is inevitable, this is clearly not so. Scientific proof, as well as my own experiences and those of my patients, provide convincing evidence that it *is* possible to stay younger while living longer.

There is a growing body of evidence that mind and body are strongly interactive. Few things happen in the body that don't start in the mind. More and more, scientists and doctors are recognizing the powerful effect of the brain on the physiology and biochemistry of the body.

For instance, feel sadness and your hormonal system goes down one biochemical path. If something in your life changes that emotion to joy, your hormonal system takes an entirely different path. Even tears of sadness have a different chemical composition than tears of joy. When you're extremely sad, your heart is bathed in chemicals that make it feel as if it's about to break. When you're full of joy, your heart is bathed by chemicals that make it feel as if it's bounding along like a playful deer.

Clearly, emotions and the workings of the physical body are closely intertwined. It is similar to the aging process: If you assume that you're old and decaying, your body will respond to that mental

1

message by slowing down and yielding quickly to the aging process. If, on the other hand, you follow the suggestions in this book and begin to treat your body as if it had many youthful, satisfying years remaining, then it will look more youthful and last much longer. So looking ten years younger and living ten years longer begins with a decision to make this book a part of your everyday life.

Beyond the foods we eat and don't eat, the supplements we take, the exercises we do and the support networks we nurture, there is the mind and the attitude toward life that helps determine how long we live. How we see our reality, negatively or positively, is important. Focusing on the negative obviously makes our inner world more negative. Conversely, focusing on the positive makes our inner world more positive and, by extension, our interactions with others as well.

## SEVEN CARDINAL RULES

In the early 1900s, people in their forties were considered old. By the 1930s, old age was considered to come about by the mid-sixties, thanks to gains in medicine, nutrition, and fitness. Currently, life expectancy has grown to early seventies for men and late seventies for women. By following the recommendations in this book, you can live into your eighties and even nineties:

### 1. Take Care of Your Body

Young adulthood, twenty years ago, was considered to be between 18 and 22. A recent Gallup poll delivered the newly emerged range of young adulthood as between 18 and 40! We're definitely living longer and staying youthful longer. This quiet revolution of longevity means that as we live longer, we take on the responsibility of caring for a body that is pioneering a new path. Such courage deserves special consideration.

### 2. Continue to Expect Ongoing Energy and Endurance

We must learn to break tradition and destructive mythologies about aging. In terms of physical strength, we can continue to expect ongo-

ing energy and endurance instead of settling into the proverbial rock-
ing chair. At age 76, sportswoman Helen Borchard of New York City
was still playing nine holes of golf before lunch, nine holes after
lunch during the summer, then tennis and swimming every Tuesday
and Thursday with her friends. At night she was busy working toward
a new degree, not getting to bed till 12 midnight or 1 A.M.

### 3. Continue to Enjoy Your Sex Life

A discouraging myth about sex among the aging would have them
giving up sex for the most part in the later years. The Starr-Weiner
Report questioning over 800 people between the ages of 60 and 91
revealed that 97 percent of this group enjoyed their sex lives and 75
percent considered their sex lives at least as or more enjoyable than
when they were younger.

### 4. Keep Your Lifestyle Young

It appears that remaining fit as a fiddle into those special extra ten
years has more to do with lifestyle than any intrinsic physical limitations. Consider, for example, the careers of jazz singer Maxine
Sullivan, who, at the young age of 68, made a career switch from
night-club-circuit singer to Broadway actress, winning a Tony for her
performance in My Old Friends; and Nellie Thompson, an active lob-
byist in the Florida state legislature at age 78, occasionally working
from 6 A.M. to 12 midnight.

### 5. Slow Down as Little as Possible

Making these extra ten years as healthy and fit as possible begins by
extending the fitness of our young adulthood as much as possible,
and slowing down as little as possible over the passing years. Let's
look at the example set by physical fitness expert, Marjorie Craig.
Author of the best-selling Miss Craig's 21-Day Shape-Up Program, Ms.
Craig still maintained her enviable figure at age 67 after 29 years as
a fitness expert at Elizabeth Arden's New York salon.

### 6. Maintain a Healthy Routine

Getting up at 6 A.M., Ms. Craig had her usual breakfast of one orange,
one slice of bread and one cup of coffee, then on to work for 10 half-

hour private classes each day. She'd swim every day after work, and then take a walk in the woods by her home, if time permitted.

## 7. Never Allow Yourself to Become Inactive

The elegant simplicity of an active lifestyle is in the ongoing nature of it over the passing decades, even into the 60s, 70s and 80s. One research project studied 184 healthy but inactive people over the age of 60. Part of this group began an exercise program while the other members of the group remained inactive. After two years, 13 percent of the inactive people exhibited new heart problems. Of the exercisers, only 2 percent showed such problems.

"You can start exercising at any time of your life," according to Ms. Craig. "When you begin you might have to take it slowly because your body isn't in condition, but once you learn the routine it's easy."

DAILY EXERCISE ROUTINES—THROUGHOUT LIFE. How better to have a sense of control over one's life than to be as physically fit as possible! Daily exercise routines that are enjoyable can be followed throughout life. At 65, 75, or even 85, women may have less vim and vigor, but still maintain a sufficient store of energy to continue to enjoy whatever physical exercise they choose.

Whenever I run my 5K or 10K Saturday morning races, I always keep an eye out for senior runners. If possible, I create an opportunity to chat with these inspiring individuals. In their 60s, 70s and 80s, these wonderful women continue to run competitively, and in the process, gain the benefits of "successful aging." Their sense of control over their own lives is much greater because of their enhanced physical strength and endurance. This in turn adds years to life, as well as adding life to years. According to Yale psychologist Judith Rodin, "Control is more likely to affect health than health is to affect control."

## WOMEN'S LIFE EXPECTANCY IS GREATER NOW THAN EVER BEFORE

But how long can women remain competitive runners? The simple answer is—ten years longer. A more thoughtful answer has to deal with the question—ten years longer than what? Although my promise in this book is ten years longer than if you didn't follow the recommendations I propose, there is growing evidence that ten years of longer life may be a modest expectation.

Writing in the *Journal of Human Evolution*, Richard Cutler has calculated the mean lifetime potential (MLP) of various animal species, based on rate of development, length of reproductive period and brain size. According to Cutler's calculations, the MLP of humans is 110 years.

This surprisingly high figure is in rough agreement with that of Kenneth Manton of Duke University who analyzed extensive U. S. Census data to determine that the "life endurance" of Americans is 114 years.

And finally, citing data from the Census Bureau, Paul Siegel and Cynthia Teauber report similar findings: "If the average annual rates of decrease in age-specific death rates recorded in the years since 1968 continue to prevail in the coming 65 years (to 2050), the average life expectation would approximate 100 in that year."

## Life "Begins" at Sixty-five

Now you may more easily understand why the title of this chapter is: "Growing Old, Staying Young." Living ten years longer is no mere fantasy. Instead of living into our 60s, 70s or 80s, we can look forward to even more years of "successful aging"—up to 100 years or more, according to the above-mentioned research.

Some accounts of the longevity of individuals in the (then) Soviet Caucasus are mind-boggling. Perhaps in a few cases, the truth was even stretched. But the number of studies of large groups and the actuarial projections based on solid historical facts gleaned from national data banks, all point to longevity beyond our normal expectations. For example, an individual claiming to be 138 years old was found to be exaggerating the truth. When the proper documentation was uncovered, it turned out that this person was merely 101. Merely?! Not bad, even though this person exaggerated a bit.

Here in the United States, where official records are highly reliable, the *Guinness Book of Records* listed Margaret Skeete as the oldest living person in America. Her age was verified from an 1880 census listing her as a two-year-old at the time. At her 115th birthday on October 27, 1993, Ms. Skeete appeared unimpressed by her exceptional longevity. She died seven months later in May of 1994, in Radford, Virginia.

According to the *Guinness Book* at the time of this writing, the oldest person in the world is 120-year-old Jeanne Calment of France. Apparently, the old folks in the mountains of Caucasus haven't bothered to write the people at the *Guinness Book*. They'd make Ms. Calment look young in comparison. Then again, they've got other things to do.

But what really count are the studies that focus on large groups rather than accounts of individuals. In his book *Who Shall Live?* Victor Fuchs compares two adjacent states—Utah and Nevada—with similar climates and topography. He found that, despite the similarities, deaths from cirrhosis and lung cancer were two to six times higher in Nevada than in Utah. The reason is that Utah is populated largely by Mormons, whose religion forbids smoking and alcohol. Across the U.S., Mormons live 30 percent longer than their fellow Americans. So this statistic alone would suggest that you can hope to live at least ten years longer just by following the suggestions from my chapter on smoking. Following the remaining suggestions on nutrition, fitness, and so on, should virtually *guarantee* the additional ten years I promise.

## "LONGEVITY POTENTIAL" TEST

To determine where you presently are in the process of gaining ten more years of happy, healthy living, take the following test.

Each area of your longevity potential is covered over 20 items. There is a 5-point scale so that you can make the most accurate estimate of your own lifestyle. If for any reason you cannot answer a certain item, just circle '3' in the middle of the scale. For example, if you have no idea what your cholesterol level is for Item 9, just circle '3.' Then add up all the circled responses to get your total. The test will allow you to compare your score to those of your friends or others in your family.

After you've finished reading the book and have had a chance to start making changes, you can take this test again to see how much you've changed. Take the test every 3 months or so to see how you're doing. That way, you can monitor your progress over time.

# "LONGEVITY POTENTIAL" TEST

1. Do you feel in charge of your life or a victim of circumstances?

| in charge | | | | victim |
|---|---|---|---|---|
| 5 | 4 | 3 | 2 | 1 |

2. In general, do you feel stressed or relaxed?

| relaxed | | | | stressed |
|---|---|---|---|---|
| 5 | 4 | 3 | 2 | 1 |

3. In general, do you feel confident or overwhelmed?

| confident | | | overwhelmed | |
|---|---|---|---|---|
| 5 | 4 | 3 | 2 | 1 |

4. In general, do you choose to eat high-fat foods (cakes, cookies, beef, sauces) or low-fat foods (pasta, vegetables, rice, fruit)?

| low-fat | | | high-fat | |
|---|---|---|---|---|
| 5 | 4 | 3 | 2 | 1 |

5. Have your attempts at dieting ended up with weight gain instead of loss?

| no | | | | yes |
|---|---|---|---|---|
| 5 | 4 | 3 | 2 | 1 |

6. Do you consistently take a vitamin supplement?

| yes | | | | no |
|---|---|---|---|---|
| 5 | 4 | 3 | 2 | 1 |

7. Do you enjoy a healthy sex life?

| yes | | abstaining | | no |
|---|---|---|---|---|
| 5 | 4 | 3 | 2 | 1 |

8. Do you manage to exercise three or more times a week?

| 3 or more | | once a week | | never |
|---|---|---|---|---|
| 5 | 4 | 3 | 2 | 1 |

9. Is your cholesterol level over 200?

| 140 | | 200 | | 240 |
|---|---|---|---|---|
| 5 | 4 | 3 | 2 | 1 |

10. How many cigarettes a day do you smoke?

| 0 | 10 | 20 | 30 | 40+ |
|---|---|---|---|---|
| 5 | 4 | 3 | 2 | 1 |

11. How many ounces of alcohol per day do you consume?

| 0-2 | 3 | 4-5 | 6 | 7+ |
|---|---|---|---|---|
| 5 | 4 | 3 | 2 | 1 |

12. Do you make use of sunscreen to avoid exposure to the sun?

| always | usually | sometimes | rarely | never |
|---|---|---|---|---|
| 5 | 4 | 3 | 2 | 1 |

13. Are your relationships supportive?

| yes | | | | no |
|---|---|---|---|---|
| 5 | 4 | 3 | 2 | 1 |

14. Do you generally communicate well at a deeper level?

| always | | | | never |
|---|---|---|---|---|
| 5 | 4 | 3 | 2 | 1 |

15. Do you consider this stage in your life as good or better than any previous ones?

| yes | | | | no |
|---|---|---|---|---|
| 5 | 4 | 3 | 2 | 1 |

16. Do you usually get the medical check-ups suggested by doctors?

| yes | | | | no |
|---|---|---|---|---|
| 5 | 4 | 3 | 2 | 1 |

17. Do you usually see a doctor if you sense something may be wrong?

| yes | | | | no |
|---|---|---|---|---|
| 5 | 4 | 3 | 2 | 1 |

18. Do you find yourself worrying much of the time?

| no | | | | yes |
|---|---|---|---|---|
| 5 | 4 | 3 | 2 | 1 |

19. Do you enjoy being sensitive to others' needs or do you feel others should be more sensitive to your feelings?

| sensitive to others | | | others sensitive to me | |
|---|---|---|---|---|
| 5 | 4 | 3 | 2 | 1 |

20. Do you feel you have a sense of purpose in life, or do you often feel lost and confused?

| purpose | | | lost and confused | |
|---|---|---|---|---|
| 5 | 4 | 3 | 2 | 1 |

## SCORING

Total your points. \_\_\_\_\_

| | Points |
|---|---|
| Likely to increase your lifespan by ten years. | 90–100 |
| Likely to increase your lifespan by five years. | 80– 89 |
| Unlikely to change your lifespan. | 70– 79 |
| Read this book carefully. | 60– 69 |
| Make this book your constant companion. | 50– 59 |
| Call your doctor immediately! | 40– 49 |
| Have you completed your will? | 20– 39 |

# CHRONOLOGICAL AGE VS. BIOLOGICAL AGE

Two researchers, William Evans and Irwin Rosenberg (authors of *Biomarkers*), studied 623 individuals who "tested biologically older than their chronological or calendar age—many by ten years or more." Within four months, these subjects were able to reduce their body age by over eight years. They looked younger, reached ideal weight, and reduced the number and depth of facial wrinkles. They felt better, with more energy and enthusiasm for life. The result of their research: "People in their fifties and sixties are as able to lower their body ages as people in their thirties and forties." More than 96 percent of the subjects ended up reducing their biological ages.

## Keep Your Life as Stress-Free as Possible

One of the key factors that contributes to aging is the amount of stress in your life and how you deal with it. Grief and depression are often the precursors to such autoimmune diseases as rheumatoid arthritis. Even cancer is affected by the emotions. In his popular book, *Anatomy of an Illness*, Norman Cousins was able to cure himself of terminal cancer by exposing himself to as much humor as he could get a hold of, whether through watching funny movies or reading humorous books.

Dr. Hans Selye, the pioneer of stress research, was able to cure himself of a type of cancer by committing himself to "try to squeeze as much from life now as you can . . . because I'm a fighter, and cancer provided me with the biggest fight of my life." Although doctors gave him less than one year to live, he went on to live a full and productive life for another 10 years, dying a natural death at age 75. In the words of Dr. Bernie Siegel, author of the best-selling *Love, Medicine and Miracles*, "Exceptional patients refuse to be victims. They educate themselves and become specialists in their own care."

# PROFILE OF A WOMAN WELL OVER ONE HUNDRED

Mary Sims Elliott, 104 years of age at the time of this writing, lives in Athens, Georgia, and is one of the subjects of research scientists studying those who have passed the age of 100. According to these experts, over three quarters of such long-living individuals are women with dominant personalities and good coping skills. In addition, they share the following characteristics:

1. Only 1 percent smoke.

2. About half consume at least some alcohol.

3. Few suffer from depression, though it is otherwise common among the elderly.

Scientists have studied the lifestyles of the long-lived individuals of the Checheno-Ingush Republic in the Northern Caucasus. Those living in the mountains had less than one-tenth the number of strokes and about one-tenth the number of heart attacks as those living down in the plains. There was six times as much hypertension in the plains as in the mountains, and twice as much as in the foothills.

Why were the mountain folk so much healthier? Those living in the mountains were much more likely to be in a "good mood" or positive mental disposition. These were individuals who lived to 90 or more. Eighty-three percent of these long-lived mountain folk were pastoral and agricultural workers living "an unhurried pace of life."

One outstanding example was Khfaf Lazuria, 139 years old at the time of the study, living in her native village, Kutol, in the then-Soviet Republic of Abkhasia. Reputed to be the oldest woman alive, Khfaf was a bright, affectionate, sprightly woman with a fine sense of humor who could still thread a needle without the aid of eyeglasses.

Khfaf had first married at the age of 40 and still managed to outlive four husbands. Her fourth marriage took place at the relatively young age of 108. She continued working and even at the age of 128 could still gather as much as 25 kilos of harvested tea, serving as a model for less efficient workers.

At the age of 139, she continued to keep active, taking care of all her own needs, caring for a good-sized garden and playing with her great-grandchildren. The next year Khfaf finally got her well-deserved 15 minutes of fame. All the way from Moscow came a delegation replete with TV cameras in order to film this extraordinary woman on the occasion of her 140th birthday. When she was asked if she could still dance, Khfaf hardly hesitated but went immediately into a jig, shifting her cane from hand to hand, alternately waving each hand as the dance required.

Unfortunately, death eventually claims us all. The next year, after admitting to not feeling well, Khfaf selected her own grave site not far from that of her late husband, and died peacefully on February 14, 1975.

The home where she was living with her stepson and his youngest son and family was not the same for quite a while. Khfaf was well-liked and respected by all who knew her. Despite her age, Khfaf had been listed as the head of household and maintained a strong sense of pride in her relationships with all her kinfolk. Her family mourned her death for many months.

## The Importance of Support Systems

Kinship, family closeness, and good friends provide the basis for critical support systems as you age. Marriage, family, and old friends provide the continuity of supportive ongoing relationships.

It may not be essential to be married to enjoy a longer life, but a reliable group of friends, some elders you can count on for sage advice, and younger people who respect and appreciate your opinions certainly help.

## Stay Stressed, but Avoid Distress

According to Hans Selye, stress "accelerates the rate of aging through the wear and tear of daily living." Khfaf Luzuria and her compatriots age at a very slow pace. Part of the reason is the minimal amount of stress in their lives. However, minimal stress does not mean inactivity and passivity. It means the absence of *distress*, as Selye uses the term. Healthy stress, as in sexual excitement, social excitement and physical challenge is an essential part of life. In this way, you want to stay stressed as you grow older. It's the *distress* you want to avoid—fear, anxiety, alienation, depression.

One important way to keep challenging stress from becoming *distress* is to have the support of close friends and family. Here are three ways your family and friends will help increase your longevity:

1. *Develop a relationship with someone you can talk to and trust with your innermost feelings and thoughts.* Have at least one person in whom you

can confide the deepest, darkest secrets of your life as an essential starting point. If you can't find such a person, you might want to talk to a counselor or therapist on a regular basis.

2. *Get involved in a social group.* It's important to feel accepted and appreciated by at least one social group, be it a church group, a social group or a professional society.

3. *To get rid of anxiety, be honest.* Finally, it's important to be honest with yourself. "To thine own self be true," wrote Shakespeare, and you can be false to no other human. By being honest with yourself, and fostering a relationship of honesty and integrity with others, fear and anxiety become exceedingly rare companions. With less fear and anxiety, there is less distress on the inner workings of the body, and therefore a healthier immune system and a longer life.

Staying younger as you grow older involves being able to depend on others and having others depend on you in a supportive network.

The incredible longevity among the long-living residents of the Caucasus is attributed to a large extent to their support systems and relatively stress-free life. In a group studied in the mountains of Daghestan, there were over ten times as many people over the age of 90 as there were in the cities of the plains below. At the time of the study, there were 187 nonagenarians (people whose age is in the nineties) for every 10,000 in the mountain areas and only 17 in the cities below—more than ten times the number of folks over the age of 90. In this study, the nonagenarians in the mountains of the Northern Caucasus were far more active and "more interested in life" than their counterparts in the cities below.

Sula Benet, who lived among these people for months at a time, met a 107-year-old man who said, "I am not old yet. I am in good health and working. I will be all right yet for a long time to come." After meeting scores of such long-living people, Benet concluded: "In the Caucasus, people feel that as long as they are in good health, working, and functioning in their social roles, they are not old."

Even fertility and child-rearing can go on into maturity. Agsha Bartzitz got married at the age of 35 and had her sixth child at the age of 47. At the age of 104, she was still doing well in her village of Blaburkhua, keeping house and feeding the chickens.

Late menopause is part of the longevity pattern in this culture. Over a three-year period, according to noted gerontologist Ramazan Alikishiev, 1,000 babies were born to women over 50 and even as old as 60. Apparently, Abkhasian doctors report that it is not at all uncommon for women of age 50 to 55 to give birth. There is an Abkhasian saying: "From mature parents come well-formed children."

Closer to home, Dr. S. Antinori of Rome, Italy has been helping postmenopausal women become pregnant and give birth. On a segment of "60 Minutes" broadcast on May 8, 1994, Dr. Antinori was shown with one of his patients, a 63-year-old woman, the oldest woman in the world to give birth. He extracted an egg from a younger woman, had it fertilized by his patient's 65-year-old husband and implanted it in her womb.

Another of Dr. Antinori's patients was Holland's oldest woman to give birth at the age of 56. Another egg-implant case, she and her 62-year-old husband are the proud parents of a bright and active little girl.

But these cases do not hold a candle to our friends in the Caucasus who have babies up to age 60 *without* egg implants. There must be something about the culture there that accounts for such long-life patterns, because it certainly isn't genetics. The gene pool in the Caucasus is extremely diverse, comprising over ten different ethnic groups.

## SECRETS FOR LONG LIFE

Part of the secret of this stress-free society is the socially supportive aspect of sharing meals. According to author Benet, "Feasts are occasions for peace making with enemies, establishing friendships, and creating good will. Past differences are often resolved, new relationships are formed, and discordant elements are brought into harmony with the well-ordered structure of living so important to the Caucasian people." At such feasts, the eldest are given the seats of highest honor, while the young "stand around the table in readiness to serve the needs of the adults."

How different from our own North-American culture, where the elderly are seen as unproductive, inflexible, and senile. According to the Pulitzer Prize-winning book, *Why Survive? Being Old in America*, by Dr. Robert Butler, older people (yet certainly younger than 90!) are considered uninteresting and condemned to a socially limited lifestyle. "There is . . . a greater debasement, a debasement based on loss of self-esteem, of significant social roles, and of a sense of importance."

## Create the Conditions of Support in Your Own Life

I myself have considered moving to China when I reach my golden years. There, old age is revered, and respect grows with the passing years—just the opposite of North America. But a more practical approach for most of us would be to take a lesson from these cross-cultural comparisons. By building close and supportive networks into our social structures, we can take responsibility to create the conditions for our own increase of lifespan by ten youthful years.

A study of 7,000 California residents revealed that those with smaller social networks were two to three times more likely to die in a nine-year mortality study than those with larger social networks. If we understand that larger social networks provide a more stress-free world for us to enjoy our lives, it is easy to see how such psychological factors can influence our physical health.

## Develop a Take-Charge Attitude

Staying young requires an optimistic, take-charge attitude that gives you a sense of control over your life and your physical health. Frustration and stress result when you begin to feel that you have little control over your life. If you see yourself as in charge of your life and in control, you feel strong, capable and confident. If, on the other hand, you experience the events of your life as beyond your control, you feel more and more frustrated and stressed. The sense of helplessness that follows can lead to pessimism, and can shorten your life. So living ten years longer requires a take-charge attitude in which there is a sense of control over most of life's challenges.

Research has shown that feeling out of control over a period of time can lead to a weak immune system, and life-threatening illness.

On the other hand, feeling strong, in charge, and optimistic can result in a stronger immune system.

To explore this very specific relationship between optimism and function of the immune system, scientists at the University of Pennsylvania studied 47 individuals between the ages of 60 and 90. They took blood samples from these people and examined the ratio of "helper" cells to "suppressor" cells, a high ratio indicating a healthy immune function. The results: The higher the degree of healthy optimism, the stronger the immune system.

As further proof that a confident, optimistic approach to life boosts the immune system, another scientist found that optimistic college students were less frequently ill than pessimistic students (3.7 days versus 8.6 days) and had to visit their doctors less frequently (once a year versus 3.6 times a year). Is it any wonder that Norman Cousins was able to cure himself of a debilitating collagen disease by watching funny movies from his hospital bed!

How do you begin to choose a path of self-confidence and optimism that will lead to a longer life?

1. *Choose a supportive environment.* Choosing successful experiences in childhood would be an excellent start. But since we can't go back in time, where do we start now? We do so by choosing to be with people who are supportive and encouraging. It's been illustrated that students often react to teachers' expectations of success or failure. We often respond to others' subtly expressed expectations of us, even as adults. By choosing a supportive environment, we set the stage for self-improvement and a growing sense of confidence.

2. *Find a partner.* For starters, look for a close, trusted partner with whom to share your new adventure. This individual will offer encouragement with realistic, honest feedback as you pioneer this new path. If both of you decide to begin together, all the better. You can be each other's support and feedback system all rolled into one good partner.

3. *Find your master.* Another way to increase self-confidence is to choose an area on which to focus, and then choose models or mentors who can teach you by example or by instruction. You can choose to learn from those you already know, or if that individual isn't available in person, you can watch from a distance (as in classes or lec-

tures), obtain videotapes of her or read about her. Having a mentor is extremely helpful.

4. *Take action.* Once you've chosen an area in which to focus, whether it be a social skill, a healthier way of eating, or an athletic or intellectual skill, then take action. You may not be as comfortable as you'd like when starting a new behavior, but here are a few tips to help you along the way.

5. *Give yourself big rewards for small steps at first.* Start slowly. Take little steps at first. Give yourself (or one another) big rewards for small beginning steps. Think of an automobile engine. First gear moves slowly but takes a lot of fuel. By the time you get to fourth gear and the car's already picked up momentum, it takes much less fuel to move quickly over greater distances. If overdrive is available, the car speeds along with minimal fuel consumption. So give yourself (or one another) a lot of fuel in terms of reward and encouragement during the beginning phases. As time goes by and small successes lead to larger ones, you can ease up on the need for reward and encouragement and just allow time to share success stories and look for the new challenges.

6. *Breaking the ice—fake it till you make it.* One of the challenges in beginning a new skill or habit is that it doesn't feel familiar. Of course not! If it did, you wouldn't be exploring new territory. At this point, many feel that since the new behavior doesn't feel familiar or comfortable, then it's experienced as phony—not the "true me." This is often used as an excuse to avoid trying this new experiment. "It's just not me," you might find yourself saying. "It's not in my personality."

Well, here's where the nuts and bolts of self-confidence come in. It's your decision to choose something new—to improve your life—that can now prevail, to replace poor habits that lead to disappointment and a discouraging sense of helplessness. So if you have to "fake it until you make it," then do so. If you're so overweight that jogging makes you bounce all over and embarrasses you, then walk at first in a mall or airport instead of at a track or spa. If crowds scare you and you decide to become more social, then attend low-key social gatherings at first, concentrating on one person at a time. Learn to do simple things such as developing a firm handshake while smiling and making eye contact. Allow yourself to be curious about this new person and questions of interest will flow naturally. Virtually all people enjoy talking about themselves to someone who has a genuine interest. Don't forget to give yourself (and each other) lots of credit for these simple yet challenging steps.

7. *Master each step thoroughly before moving on.* Stay with the first, early steps a bit longer than you'd like. Don't move ahead too quickly. Allow yourself sufficient success with the beginning steps until you become slightly bored with them. That means you've mastered them thoroughly; they're no longer the challenges they once were. Now you're ready to move ahead to the next level of challenge, whether that means walking/jogging on a track or telling a single joke to the new people you meet after you've chatted about yourselves. Enjoy your mastery of each beginning step before moving on. In acquiring self-confidence, moving slowly is much more efficient than speeding ahead before you've mastered the step at hand.

8. *Keep track of your progress.* Keep aware of your progress in some systematic fashion. The best way to do this is to keep some sort of chart, using some measure of progress. It's amazing how rewarding it is to actually see your progress in chart form, so you can actually count your successes. Success breeds upon itself, as does failure. So even if your successful steps are small (as they should be), it's important to be able to see these successes at a glance.

### Lowering My Own Blood Pressure

At one point, in my own self-determination for better health, I decided to try garlic pills to see if I could successfully lower my blood pressure. I had read anecdotes indicating that this could be done, although strong medical proof was lacking. Rather than waiting for more research, I decided to try my own experiment using myself as the subject. I borrowed a blood pressure cuff to record my progress.

This was in the summer of '91. I started recording my blood pressure ten days before starting on the garlic pills. I began taking the garlic pills on the first of June. The average reading for the days May 21 through 31 was 126/87. Then I started the pills. For the first half of June my reading went down on the diastolic side only, from 87 to 82. For the second half of June, both systolic and diastolic went down to 116/74. I continued the pills and the recording through July. The first half of July, the average reading was 119/78, the second half,

115/78. I was satisfied now that the garlic pills had helped my blood pressure to go down about 10 points. This doesn't mean that it'll work that way for everyone, but at least I was satisfied that it helped me. The importance of the charting was in its graphic representation of success. I continue taking garlic pills to this day. There's nothing like looking at a chart full of successes when you start getting discouraged, whether you're charting blood pressure, miles walked/jogged or jokes told.

9. *Learn from your mistakes.* Another way to enhance self-confidence is to manage your emotions. By that, I mean to understand your feelings, both through introspection and by getting feedback from trusted friends. When frustrated and angry, acknowledge these feelings initially and then let them go. Replace them with a curiosity as to how events led to the frustration. What could you have done to avert failure? Once you discover the answer to this question, don't blame yourself but, instead, consider yourself the wiser and more able to glean success from similar circumstances in the future.

10. *Stay honest.* The healthiest communication style for enhancing self-confidence is assertive honesty. Holding back on the expression of one's needs is unhealthy and actually life-threatening. Life expectancy is strongly influenced by having a resilient and resourceful psychological makeup. The more self-expressive we are, the more self-confidence we bring about in our lives, and the longer we can expect to live.

11. *Choose your own lifestyle.* Across the ages there have been periods when individuals have had more self-confidence than others, and it is during these "eras of personal power" that people add years to their lives. In the Middle Ages of Europe, for example, when the opportunities for individual expression and personal choice were at a minimum, life expectancy was low. On the other hand, as we currently experience a period of growing personal power and individual rights, the normal lifespan is growing in years. One of the components of this trend to longer life is the opportunity for women to choose their own lifestyles, including different habits of eating and fitness.

Despite the large amounts of money spent by the food industry on advertising fast foods and snacks that are too fat, too sweet, and generally unhealthy, more and more women are choosing to decrease their consumption of such foods and the trend seems to be in the direction of a healthier eating lifestyle. Personal confidence in this case means choosing healthier food despite a cultural influence in the opposite direction. The more in control of their lives women feel, the more they can express themselves, the more their rights are protected and the longer they will live.

12. *Give away your success.* Finally, become a giver in your area of success. There's no better way to lock in success than to share it with others. If you've discovered something that contributes to your health, let others know about it. If you're becoming more physically fit, offer to assist someone else in her struggle. If you're gaining in social confidence, support those who are as shy as you once were.

## TEN-POINT LIFESTYLE PROGRAM

1. Find a friend or family member with whom to share your lifestyle changes.

2. Share this book with your new partner.

3. Take the time to support one another.

4. Learn these four affirmations on which you can meditate:

   a. "My entire body feels ten years younger and I feel as sexy as ever."

   b. "My choices in lifestyle, grooming and skin care allow me to look ten years younger."

   c. Choose an affirmation of your own that relates to your love life. Think about what you'd most like to have to feel better and focus on that. For example, "I choose to enjoy great sex with my partner by creating the right opportunities for that," or "Every day I choose to make a positive difference in my lover's life."

   d. Choose an affirmation of your own relating to a personal goal, such as losing a certain number of pounds, or increasing your distance on the jogging trail. This should be a goal that you can easily measure and that is fairly easily attainable. For example, "I can feel myself becoming thinner and expect to lose two pounds by next month," or "I can feel my body becoming more fit and expect to be able to keep up with my jogging partner by the end of the month."

5.  Spend at least one-half hour a day relaxing with your lover and sharing your best self in an emotionally intimate way.

6.  Make a personal commitment to three hours per week of your favorite exercise in any combination you like.

7.  For the next six months, select one chapter from this book and make that chapter your companion for the month. Read it, reflect on it, and try its suggestions on for size. At the beginning of the next month, select any other chapter. Don't  necessarily go in chronological order. Select the chapter that appeals to you most at the time.

8.  Forge ahead on all fronts slowly but consistently.

9.  Compare notes with your partner and support one another's progress. Focus on improvements in health and appearance. Celebrate your successes together: a healthy meal at your favorite restaurant, great seats at the theater, a weekend away.

10. After six months or so, whenever you feel you've achieved sub-stantial change, choose your own way of sharing your success with others, such as volunteering to help others less fortunate than yourself, coaching at your local high school, teaching, or writing. There's nothing to lock in your hard-earned successes like sharing them with others.

When all is shared and done, you too can look ten years younger and live ten years longer. All it takes is a decision—one that can change the entire course of your life and your health.

> *"It isn't until you come to a spiritual understanding of who you are—*
> *not necessarily a religious feeling, but deep down, the spirit within—*
> *that you can begin to take control."*
>
> **—Oprah Winfrey**

# DR. RYBACK'S
## ANTIAGING FOOD PLAN

CHAPTER 2

$N$ote the wisdom of Estelle Wolf at age 94: "I try to eat nourishing meals. I don't eat junk food. I like to cook. I try to eat a variety of foods. A dinner might be a piece of meat or fish, fresh vegetables, salad and then fruit for dessert."

Diets don't work, as most of us know by now. Only when we can make long-lasting changes that feel comfortable will we successfully manage our weight problems. Fun ways to exercise will stick, according to Sheryl Marks Brown, Executive Director of the American Council on Exercise. Crash diets and fanatical exercise regimes just don't work.

According to the latest research involving a 14-year study of over 100,000 women, even small weight gains in adulthood significantly increase the risk of developing heart disease.

Eating is something most of us do at least three times a day. If we control this ongoing activity, we can do more to look younger and live longer than by doing any other single activity in our lives. Almost on a daily basis, we read about more and more research findings that inform us of the importance of choosing the right foods.

### The Natural Power in Fruits and Vegetables

Recent reports indicate that just by eating a couple of generous servings of such vegetables as carrots and broccoli and such fruits as apricots and cantaloupe, we can:

1. help prevent cancer;

2. decrease the risk of developing angina; and

3. prevent coronary heart disease in general.

So you see, it doesn't take all that much effort. It's just a matter of educating yourself and making some wise choices. In this chapter, we'll explore the basics of intelligent nutrition along with the use of vitamin and mineral supplements, and offer sound research to back these findings. The basics are very simple. And in all likelihood, you've heard much of it before. But here we bring it all together so that we can minimize the confusion and gain control over what we put in our mouths.

### How Each Diet Makes Us Fatter

As we lose weight through dieting, fat cells do not shrink in number but merely in size. Once we give up on our diet, those little fat cells soak up all the fat they can to regain their normal size and if we continue our fat intake beyond that, then additional fat cells will add to our bulk. It appears that we can *increase* the number of fat cells *easily* but we cannot *decrease* their number. This helps us understand how we get fatter and fatter with each successive diet.

So, even though diets promise, and can deliver weight losses of four or more pounds per week, such diets are effective only for a week or so, and then cause either a very frustrating plateau or a rebound effect to sabotage any remaining ounces of motivation.

### "Yo-Yo" Dieting

By now, most of us are familiar with "yo-yo" dieting: lose X number of pounds and then, when we relax our crash diets, regain X + Y number of pounds. Repeat this a couple of times a year, and we're on our way to chronic obesity.

One of my patients, a teacher in her late 30s, is a prime example. Joan, 5'1" tall, could lose as much as 40 pounds when going on a diet, but as soon as she began eating normally, she'd lose control and gain back what she lost and then some.

When she first came to my office, Joan broke down in tears and told me: "Dr. Ryback, a number of years ago, I went on a diet and lost

20 pounds; then when I began eating normally, I just lost control. I couldn't help myself. I was using both hands to stuff food into my mouth as fast as I could. I regained the 20 pounds I had lost and put on another 5.

"The next year I went on a diet again and was able to lose 25 pounds. But when I ended the diet, the same thing happened, only this time I regained another 40 pounds. The following year, the same pattern occurred. And so it went! I'm now up to 170 pounds. You've got to help me!"

Here is a prime example of yo-yo dieting. Joan went from 125 pounds to 105 pounds (X = 20 pounds lost.) Then she regained the lost weight plus an additional 5 pounds. (X + Y = 20 + 5 or 25 pounds)

The next year, she lost 25 pounds but regained 40 (X + Y = 25 + 15). The following year, she lost 40 pounds, but gained back 45 (X + Y = 40 + 5).

This kept up until she reached 170 pounds—quite a lot of poundage for an otherwise petite 5'1" school teacher. Obviously, crash diets don't work!

It should be clear by now that dramatic or yo-yo dieting just plain doesn't work. More than that, it's downright dangerous. When a dramatic attempt at dieting ends, more weight is gained than was lost and usually in the worst possible place—around the belly. The ongoing Framingham Heart Study has shown that those whose weight fluctuated the most over a 20-year period had a higher death rate than those whose weight fluctuated the least. So don't attempt dramatic diets. Just gradually teach yourself to eat less fat in the foods you do eat and learn to enjoy combinations of fruits and vegetables more and more.

## TEN ANTIAGING NUTRITION BASICS

My antiaging food plan demands complete commitment and a full realization and acceptance of the fact that, inevitably, there will be setbacks. To do it right, be absolutely sure you don't overlook the following ten basic rules:

1. *Set reasonable goals.* Be wary of standard height/ weight tables. What is really important is the ratio of muscle to fat. A muscular woman may appear overweight according to standard tables. A woman who is out of shape may yet appear to be the right weight, with the wrong muscle-to-fat ratio.

A more efficient standard for women would be for body fat to be 20 to 27 percent of total body weight. To best determine your body fat (other than through hydrodensitometry or underwater weighing), have someone with experience measure you with skin calipers. Try a good health club or your local university's department of physical education, exercise physiology, or nutrition.

2. *Don't lose sight of reality.* **Important:** Slow and gradual weight loss works. Sudden and dramatic losses in weight don't work. The body needs to adjust to weight loss if the loss is to be even some-what permanent. Ideally, you should plan to lose about one or two pounds per week. It's much better to take a year to lose 50 pounds and keep it off in a healthy manner than to impress yourself and others with a dramatic loss that just comes back to haunt you and shame you to your friends. Best of all, it's much easier to do it the healthier way.

The dramatic ads you see in the magazines and on TV to shed pounds quickly and effortlessly in weeks (or even days) are false and pernicious. The only part of your being that will end up permanently lighter will be your wallet. These ads take advantage of the fact that it is easy to lose weight in the beginning of any diet, but this is main-ly due to water loss.

3. *Convert poor nutritional habits to good ones.* Discover your patterns of eating by keeping an eating journal. For a couple of weeks, keep note of 1.) what you eat, 2.) how much, 3.) when, 4.) where, 5.) what you're doing at the time, and 6. how you're feeling at the time.

The answers to these questions will help you discover the pat-tern of your eating habits. Only then will you learn how to change these patterns so that you can gain control over the details of your life that determine your particular eating habits.

You may be surprised how much certain places (kitchen, restau-rant), times (noon, dinner time), activities (watching TV or movies), or feelings (loneliness, anger) determine your eating habits. Instead of letting these circumstances decide, you can now master your eating habits by controlling some of these circumstances, at least some of the time. You can gain more control over these circumstances over time just as you can learn any other skill—with *attention* and *intention*.

4. *Follow a balanced, low-fat food plan.* Make sure to eat a variety of foods from the basic food groups. Whenever possible, choose carbohydrates over fats. Eat lots of fruits, vegetables, and grains. This makes you feel full and provides good nutrition at a most reasonable cost.

5. *Avoid high-fat foods.* Do your best to avoid high-fat foods such as red meat and its by-products:

- hamburger, meatloaf
- hot dogs, luncheon meats

as well as:

- whole milk and cheese
- baked goods such as cookies, cakes, doughnuts
- fried foods
- gravy and cream sauce
- most crackers and chips
- ice cream
- most nuts, especially almond, macadamia, and coconut

6. *Find the eating pattern that's comfortable for you.* The important thing here is to explore patterns of eating until you find one that feels comfortable for you and gives you a sense of mastery over your eating habits and your body weight. Otherwise, the changes you worked so hard to achieve will be short-lived.

7. *Drink water with a squeeze of lemon.* Whatever option you choose, it is essential that you drink sufficient fluids throughout the day. It's a good idea to drink about eight cups of water throughout the day, even if you drink it in the form of your favorite beverages. Keep in mind, too, that many soft drinks contain hefty measures of sugar unless they are diet drinks. A squeeze of lemon in cool water is an excellent option.

8. *Learn to limit libations.* Limit your alcohol to no more than two drinks a day.

9. *Exercise.* The best insurance against regaining the weight you've lost is to incorporate exercise into your everyday routine.

Find an activity that you can 1.) enjoy, 2.) fit into your life so that you can continue it without too much difficulty, and 3.) make sure that it's an ongoing part of your life by arranging the rest of your life around it.

Here are some helpful hints:

1. Make a routine of your exercise activity but allow for interesting changes within that routine.

2. Arrange your schedule so that you exercise the same time each day. This will help make it a permanent fixture in your life without your having to make a decision to exercise each time.

3. If you enjoy exercising alone, you can choose from: walking, jogging, swimming, weight lifting, aerobics, exercycling, hitting a ball against a backboard, and so on.

4. If you prefer socializing, enjoy any of the above with your favorite friends, or try team sports such as tennis, volleyball, and soccer. Join the local Y and see what it has to offer. If you have a lot of social frustration in your life, you might consider judo or karate.

5. If you drive to work, park a few blocks from work (and possibly save some parking fees). Walk the rest of the way to work and jog back to your car after work. Take the stairs instead of the elevator. Instead of having a three-course meal at the cafeteria, take a noontime stroll and finish it off with low-fat yogurt and fresh fruit. Then spend the rest of the afternoon enjoying how much better you feel than your associates.

10. *Create meaningful markers or milestones to celebrate your successes.* For example, for each 5, 10, or 20 pounds you lose, reward yourself with something you enjoy but wouldn't ordinarily give yourself. A theater or concert ticket, taking a close friend to one of your favorite restaurants to share a healthy meal, buying yourself an article of clothing you've wanted or a special piece of jewelry—any of these

can be an exciting reward to be anticipated to help motivate your thinner self.

## POWER BREAKFAST FOR LASTING YOUTH

According to one study at the VA Medical Center in Minneapolis, when 14 volunteers were given free rein at a buffet of munchies and snack foods, those who had eaten the highest fiber cereal for breakfast ate about 45 calories less at the buffet three and a half hours later.

A follow-up study divided volunteers into two groups. One had very high- and the other very low-fiber cereal for breakfast. At the buffet later in the day, the high-fiber group chose to eat 90 calories less than the other group. Starting the day with high-fiber cereal (with skim milk, of course) gives you a great head start. This one small step in itself with no other changes, continued over the span of a year, could result in a 10-pound weight loss.

Lasting youth and health, according to the National Academy of Sciences, is aided by incorporating at least five daily servings of vegetables and fruits, especially green and yellow vegetables and citrus fruits into your daily health plan. The Department of Health and Human Services recommends as many as eight servings. So a good start at breakfast means getting your share of power foods.

In addition to high-fiber cereal with skim milk, consider fresh fruit juice, with a cup of cottage cheese or low-fat yogurt containing some fresh fruit such as banana or pineapple. If you enjoy waffles or pancakes, top them with sliced fruit instead of syrup.

If you have no time for a sit-down breakfast, start your day with a blended fruit smoothie. Try banana along with one or two other fruits for the luxurious but low-fat creamy texture that the banana will give to it.

Another fast-breakfast idea comes all the way from China. The Chinese use rice left from the previous evening's meal and combine it with enough water to create a healthy, soup-like cereal. If you want to add more power to this exotic breakfast dish, add some sesame seeds and bits of cooked chicken or fish.

# FOODS THAT MAKE YOU OLD

Moving beyond breakfast for a general overview, the worst foods, those to avoid as much as possible, fall into four main categories:

1. Red meat and its by-products, including hamburgers, cheese-burgers, meatloaf.
2. Processed meats such as hot dogs, ham, and lunch meats.
3. Whole milk and cheese (except for low-fat cheese and yogurts).
4. Baked goods such as cookies, cakes, and doughnuts.

These foods are major sources of fat. Remember, too much fat in your body is implicated in helping to cause certain cancers, diabetes, hypertension, digestive problems, and complications in arthritis, not to mention heart disease and high serum cholesterol.

One of the factors responsible for meat's ill effects is the manner in which it is cooked or preserved. The way that hot dogs are cured, for example, contributes to cancer as does browning or charring while cooking. And the frying or broiling of meats creates carcinogens both within the meat and on the more apparent surface. Such carcinogens tend to form throughout the meat's outer third.

## Other High-fat Foods

Some less obvious high-fat foods that don't fit into the above four categories are:

1. Nuts (for example, macadamias, almonds, peanuts)
2. Fresh coconut
3. Avocado
4. Gravy and cream sauce
5. Salad dressings (unless fat-free)
6. Fried foods
7. Crackers

Another category of food that makes you old is that of processed, prepackaged microwave-ready meals. These are usually high in calories and have little fiber content. They typically (but not always) provide 30 percent or more calories from fat. They are almost always high in sodium content, as well.

Finally, a tricky category of food that makes you old: any packaged food that is labeled in some healthy fashion, yet actually doesn't live up to its claim. Some examples include: 2 percent milk advertised as "low-fat milk," which may keep us from choosing skim milk, which *does* have the power to keep us younger and healthier; prepackaged luncheon meals which boast "lean chicken" and "lean turkey," but along with the included high-fat cheese creates a very high-fat content overall. So take these "healthy" come-ons with a grain of suspicion.

# HOW FRESH FRUITS AND VEGETABLES ADD YEARS TO YOUR LIFE

Beyond vitamins and minerals, beyond fiber and carbohydrates, there's a relatively newly recognized substance that can add years to your life. These are known as *phytochemicals*. They are instrumental in helping to prevent the onset of cancer, and are stored by the hundreds in most plant foods. As a result of this discovery, the medical community is becoming more appreciative of the healthy nature of a vegetarian style of eating. More and more doctors are understanding the benefits of fruits and vegetables in adding healthy years to your life.

Over 12 million Americans now consider themselves vegetarians, but within this large group are smaller groupings, based on the degree of dedication to this style of nutrition. Here's how they break down.

Most of these 12 million fall into the category known as *semi-vegetarians*. They eat no red meat for the most part, but occasionally eat chicken and other fowl.

*Lacto-ovo-vegetarians* eat no meat at all, not even fowl, but will eat animal products such as milk and eggs, unlike the *lacto-vegetarians* who eat no eggs, or the *vegans* who eat no eggs and no milk products.

Many in the larger group who consider themselves vegetarians will nonetheless eat red meat, but very occasionally, and work toward minimizing their consumption of any kind of meat or fish. This seems to be the trend in society at large; moving toward less meat and more fruits and vegetables, at least among those who are mindful of adding years to their lives.

## How to Fill Yourself Up and Still Stay Thin

You could probably eat much more than you do now without gaining weight if there were no fat or processed sugar in the foods you do eat. Such foods as fruits and vegetables and whole wheat foods free of fat would likely fill you up before they'd make you fat. The Food Guide Pyramid recommends a daily intake of 6 to 11 servings of some combination of bread, cereal, rice or pasta; 2 to 4 servings of fruit; 3 to 5 servings of vegetables; and lesser servings of the other food groupings, with a sparing use of fats, oils and sweets. This guide, released by the U.S. Dept. of Agriculture, is a marked reduction from previous years in its amounts of meat and dairy products.

## The Protein Myth

The essential problem with animal protein is that it is high in artery-clogging saturated fat and cholesterol. Besides that, most Americans eat more protein than they need anyway. Adult American women, for instance, eat about 30 percent more protein than they need.

Furthermore, it may come as a surprise to most of you that you don't need *any* animal protein to be healthy. You can get all the protein you need from nonmeat sources. Yet many "red-blooded" Americans think they need to have a steak a day to eat properly. Americans eat an average of 10.6 oz. of red meat a day compared to 2.24 oz. eaten daily by the Japanese, to use one comparison.

## The Magic of Drinking Water

This might be a good point to remind you again of the benefits of drinking six to eight glasses of water each day. The older we get, the more important this becomes. As we mature, we hold less cellular water, 10 to 15 percent less by age 65. More water will certainly help us look younger as our skin cells enjoy the liquid refreshment along with all other cells.

## STAY YOUNG WITH A HIGH-FIBER, LOW-FAT DIET

Losing weight with minimal deprivation can be best accomplished not by counting calories, nor by measuring out small food portions but rather by committing yourself to a high-fiber, low-fat style of eating.

Earlier, you read about the trend toward vegetarian-style eating. Medical research is proving this to be the most effective, longest-lasting approach to weight loss and staying younger.

It's not how much you eat that matters. Different women need differing amounts of food. What does matter is the *quality* of the food you eat, in terms of fat and fiber. By following the suggestions you've read so far in this chapter, you're on your way to staying younger. By avoiding high-fat meats (especially fried) and milk products (especially cheese on pizza, cheesecake, and ice cream), you're more likely to choose healthier vegetables, fruits, and grains. Not only will you look younger and live longer; you'll feel better too, with more energy and greater alertness.

Furthermore, it's much easier. Rather than having to make many small decisions about how much to deprive yourself of rich foods, you make a big decision only once: a decision to eat healthy foods. Instead of constantly being reminded of what you're missing, you learn to enjoy the healthy foods you're choosing.

A choice to eat this way automatically provides more fiber in your diet without your having to think about it. A breakfast of high-fiber cereal with skim milk topped with half a banana along with some orange juice will keep you satisfied until you can enjoy a mid-morning snack a couple of hours later. At this time you can treat yourself to whole-wheat toast or a bagel with a bit of jam or jelly or, if you're at work, a piece of your favorite fruit. For lunch, you can enjoy some pasta with vegetables and salad, making sure that any sauces or dressings are of the very low-fat variety.

The simple thing to remember: the less processed, the better! Raw vegetables and fruits are the best. Next in order: brown rice, high-fiber bread and cereal, potatoes (unhampered by butter, of course), and pasta. Fish is better than fowl, and fowl is better than red meat, which should not be marbled with fat. Skin on fowl should be avoided. (Choose white meat over dark meat, since the dark has twice as much fat as the white.)

## What to Substitute

Instead of mayonnaise, try lettuce, tomato or cucumber for moisture. Instead of potato chips, try unsalted pretzels or air-popped popcorn. Instead of ice cream, try ice milk or sorbet. And be careful of that innocent looking peanut butter—two tablespoons contain 16.2 grams of fat.

## Choosing the Right Breads

Breads can be very healthy and enjoyable, especially "designer" breads flavored with lusty garlic and dill or onions and rosemary. Look for breads that appear chewy and have big bubbles inside. They're the ones that tend to be fat-free. Avoid the ones that have a tender, cakey texture with tiny bubbles—they're full of fat. And if the bread itself is tasty, you don't need to add fatty condiments like butter or peanut butter. Ask for fat-free, whole-wheat bread and you're more likely to get a healthy dose of fiber as well. If you don't go in for "designer" breads, then your best supermarket breads are Wonder High Fiber Wheat, Roman Meal Light Oat Bran 'N' Honey, or Roman Meal Light Seven Grain, each of these at no more than 1 gram of fat and about 6 grams of fiber per serving. Your worst choice, by far, would be Sara Lee Croissant, weighing in at 6 grams of fat and merely 0.1 grams of fiber per serving. So choose your breads carefully.

## MORE CARBOS MEAN MORE ENERGY

Loretta, a 43-year-old chemist, had always been chunky, despite the fact that she's been an avid tennis player most of her adult life. She had just moved to Atlanta and was determined to make a new start in taking care of her body. Looking at her eating habits, she realized how much meat she included in her daily diet. Rather than cut down on meat, she decided to turn over a new leaf dramatically by cutting meat out of her diet completely and becoming a vegetarian. I encouraged her to follow her feelings and discussed with her the nutrient values of various beans and grains. If this path feels right for you, I encourage you as well.

By now you can see the direction in which I'm pointing you. Animal foods such as meat and eggs and whole-milk products have no place in your diet once you make a choice to live ten years longer. Only modest portions of low-fat animal foods are to be included in your new eating habits: skinless chicken or turkey breast, fish, nonfat yogurt or cottage cheese and skim milk. If you choose to avoid meat and fish altogether, then you can replace those with more complex carbohydrates such as beans, peas and lentils.

If you choose to eat meat, then your best choice of red meat is select beef tip or eye of round. Your best choice of seafood is baked or broiled flounder or sole. If you choose to eat pork, select tenderloin. If you must eat eggs, stick to egg whites or find an egg substitute to your liking.

For those who choose to give up meat, the choice of beans and grains becomes more important. Complex carbohydrates are close to being the perfect food for living ten years longer. They are the lowest fat-to-fiber-ratio foods around, giving you the most nutrition per calorie. Fresh fruits, vegetables, beans and whole grains all are complex carbohydrates. We've already discussed fruits and vegetables. Now we'll focus on beans and grains.

Aside from being almost fat-free and full of fiber, beans and grains contain amino acids which combine to provide your body with protein. They also contain a number of vitamins and minerals. Here is an overview of what a cup of some common beans offers:

|  | Black Beans | Great Northern Beans | Kidney Beans | Navy Beans |
|---|---|---|---|---|
| B6 | 0.1 mg. | 1 mg. | 0.2 mg. | 1 mg. |
| Calcium | 47 mg. | 90 mg. | 50 mg. | 95 mg. |
| Fiber | 7 g. | 9 g. | 6 g. | 9 g. |
| Iron | 4 mg. | 5 mg. | 5 mg. | 5 mg. |
| Potassium | 611 mg. | 750 mg. | 713 mg. | 790 mg. |

They also contain folic acid, magnesium, copper, zinc, manganese, and phosphorus.

For those who are concerned about the intestinal gas that some people experience from eating beans, there is a solution. Boiling beans in a large saucepan with $1/8$ teaspoon of baking soda for 10 minutes prior to cooking will solve this. Allow the beans to cool and allow to soak at room temperature in the same water for 8 to 10 hours. Then discard the water and rinse before cooking as usual.

Another method is the simple use of the commercial product known as Beano, which, when added to bean dishes, converts the indigestible sugars into readily absorbed sugars. A free sample can be obtained by calling (800) 257-8650.

If you're not used to eating beans, start slowly, until your system adapts to them.

Just like beans, grains are also low in fat and high in fiber, at least before commercial refining. They can provide a source of ongoing, constant energy, since that is stored as glycogen in the muscles. They are eaten mostly in the form of bread, pasta, cereal, and rice dishes. Since they're low fat and filling, they do much to help you keep your weight down by providing an alternative to higher-fat foods.

The trick is to choose foods made up of whole grains rather than refined forms. Whole-grain products provide *insoluble fiber*, which helps reduce the risk of colon cancer; and *soluble fiber*, which lowers blood cholesterol.

Unfortunately, most of the grains available to Americans are of the refined type. So it's important to learn more about whole grains (including the nutritious hull and germ).

Among the most common in the U.S. and one of the most nutritious is whole-wheat flour (as opposed to refined white flour). This can be found in whole-wheat bagels, breads, English muffins, pasta, waffles and bran. *Bulgur*, wheat that has been dried and cracked, can be eaten as a cereal or side dish. Cracked-wheat salad, known as *tabbouleh*, can be a nutritious alternative to white rice.

Rice, the most common grain in the world, is most commonly consumed in the U.S. in its refined, white, polished form, deprived of its protein, minerals and B vitamins. Whole-grain or brown rice is clearly the more nutritious alternative.

Rye, oats and buckwheat can be consumed in their whole grain form in breads. Pumpernickel bread is made with dark, coarse rye ground entirely from the kernel. Oats, barley, buckwheat and rye can be consumed in the form of cooked cereal, as in oatmeal, barley soup, kasha and porridge, respectively.

A relatively unknown but rising star among healthy grains is *quinoa* (pronounced *keen-wah*). The most nutritious of all grains, quinoa contains all eight amino acids, is high in vitamin A and is one of the most protein-packed grains on the planet. It can be eaten in soups, stews, pilafs and breads to which it has been added.

If you're truly committed to living ten years longer, then you can't ignore grains as a principal nutrient in your dietary lifestyle. In addition to eating them as ingredients in other dishes, you can also learn to cook them and then just mix with a favorite flavor or topping. Generally, 1 cup of grain simmered in liquid will yield 2 to $3^1/_2$ cups of a dish.

Other ways of eating grains consist of sprinkling cooked grains onto salads, or into stews or soups. Whole wheat, brown rice or quinoa can be substituted for pasta dishes for a change of pace.

The new Food Guide Pyramid recommends six servings if you don't exercise and nine to eleven servings if you do exercise. So most of us need at least twice as much as was previously recommended by nutritionists. Here are some simple ways to increase your intake of grains:

1. Instead of high-fat snacks such as cookies or candy bars, try air-popped popcorn or rice cakes.

2. Instead of a little pasta with lots of high-fat Alfredo sauce, try more pasta with low-fat marinara sauce.

3. Allow yourself thick slabs of whole-grain bread with low-fat topping instead of thin slices of bread covered with high-fat toppings.

4. Instead of one sandwich with high-fat meat or cheese, enjoy two or three sandwiches with whole-wheat bread stuffed with leafy greens, tomatoes and cucumbers.

These complex carbohydrate treats will fill you up with healthy nutrients without getting you fattened up. It's one of the secrets of getting thinner and healthier without depriving yourself. You get to enjoy your food, have more energy and live longer in better health.

## Eating Out and Staying Thin

When you eat out, you can make certain choices that will minimize fats and increase your proportion of healthier foods. Here's what to do for various ethnic restaurants.

*Chinese*: Order steamed fish and rice or scallops sauteed with vegetables instead of heavy sauces.

*Mexican*: Order steamed instead of fried tortillas. In your better restaurants, try red snapper Vera Cruz. Avoid dishes loaded with cheese or heavy sauces. Avoid fried rice.

*French*: Order grilled or poached fish or chicken breast with steamed vegetables along with salade Nicoise, with low-fat dressing on the side. Avoid heavy sauces, no matter how tempting. Instead of pastry for dessert, order fresh fruit.

*Italian*: Order pasta dishes with marinara (meatless) sauce rather than fat-laden Alfredo. Order baked chicken rather than high-fat, cheese-laden pizza.

Women can have fun eating out and still stay healthy. It just involves making the right choices to stay thinner and live longer.

# EATING FOR YOUTHFUL FLEXIBILITY

For healthy bones and flexibility, most women need about 35 percent more calcium than they typically get. Older women can be subject to the problems of osteoporosis from which they are commonly known to suffer. Women lose about one-fifth of their bone mass over the course of a lifetime. It has been reported that women who get more calcium in their diets suffer from fewer hip fractures than those who are deficient.

## Calcium for Healthy Bones and Blood Pressure

Calcium is found primarily in milk and dairy products. Since many women suffer from lactose intolerance and can't drink milk, it's important to get this vital mineral through supplementation. Calcium may be useful in keeping our blood pressure normal as well.

Calcium in the form of milk has been known for its "tranquilizing" effects for generations, though there are no scientific data to bear this out. A number of studies do, however, point to the importance of calcium in normalizing blood pressure.

Since I recommend a diet very high in fruits, vegetables, and carbohydrates (low-calorie, and high-fiber), calcium is particularly important. Although I recommend a daily intake of 1 to 1$\frac{1}{2}$ grams, a daily intake of up to 2 or 3 grams is quite safe. Incidentally, part of my calcium supplementation is in the form of flavored Tums antacid tablets, which has a very pleasant, candy-like taste and texture. I definitely don't have stomach problems—I just enjoy that safe, pleasant form of calcium carbonate.

Calcium strengthens bones more efficiently when accompanied by adequate amounts of vitamin D. Aside from exposure to sunlight, vitamin D can be obtained from fish and fortified milk. Those women who live high in the northern hemisphere where sunlight is relatively weak in the wintertime and who, at the same time, may not get sufficient amounts of fish and fortified milk can benefit from a daily supplement of 400 International Units of vitamin D.

The U.S. Food and Drug Administration recommends a daily intake of 1000 mg. of calcium. The best source is always food rather than supplements, and the foods that supply calcium are dairy products (skim milk, yogurt, fat-free mozzarella cheese), fish and shellfish, fruits, vegetables, grains and beans.

Each of the following foods will supply about 300 mg. of calcium:

2 cups of cottage cheese

2 cups of ice milk

5 oz. of salmon

1 cup of skim milk

1 cup of yogurt

In a typical day, you can easily ensure your youthful flexibility by treating yourself to a couple of glasses of skim milk, a cup of beans, some whole-wheat cereal, a cup of nonfat yogurt and 3 oz. of fish.

If, for whatever reason, you choose to take supplements instead, there are both chewable and nonchewable tablets available. There are many supplement products from which to choose. The least expensive chewables cost less than $2 per month. It's best to take calcium supplements with meals or at bedtime for best absorption. One thing to watch out for is taking calcium supplements with iron pills or multivitamins containing iron, since calcium interferes with iron absorption.

# POWER FOODS FOR LASTING YOUTH

Any food that fortifies the immune system is one that I would consider to be a "power food." With a stronger immune system, your body can defend itself more easily against aging ravages of bacterial and viral infection as well as against cancer.

Your defense system is made up of "police" cells—including B-cells, T-cells and natural killer (NK) cells—that engulf and destroy cancer cells and infecting agents. When viruses, bacteria, or cancer cells start invading your body, it is the B-*cells* that produce the antibodies to fight against them. You may have heard of the natural substance called *interferon*, which helps fight against cancer. Well, this is produced by the T-*cells*. The NK *cells* help as well to fight against cancer and viral infections.

## Power Food I: Yogurt

Yogurt has earned a fine reputation over the years as a "folk medicine" that keeps older people young. Now there's scientific evidence that it may do so by enhancing the immune function. Here's how it works: Cultures existing in regular yogurt increase the amount of interferon in the immune system by a factor of five. So, eating only two cups of yogurt daily for a period of four months will give you this added advantage.

Recent research has shown that yogurt enhances the power of NK cells to ward off cancer too, particularly lung and colon cancer.

## Power Food II: Garlic

Most of you have also heard of the supposed healing effects of garlic. It does enhance the functioning of the immune system, most specifically by stimulating the potency of T-cells.

If you don't like the effect of garlic on your social life, have no fear. You can get the same effect from odor-free garlic extract. This will make your NK cells at least twice as powerful as those who avoid garlic.

## Power Food III: Asian Shiitake Mushrooms

You'll most often find these deliciously prepared delicacies at Chinese restaurants, nestling among other exotic vegetables. But whether you eat them there or prepare them at home yourself, these wonderful mushrooms, according to a series of research studies, contain a substance called *lentinal*, which significantly increases the number of T-cells as well as the production of other cancer-fighting substances.

Lentinal can also prevent the spreading of lung cancer cells. So this exotic mushroom not only helps reduce the risk of cancer; it helps prevent it from spreading as well.

## Power Food IV: Beta-carotene in Fruits and Vegetables

Although there may be some controversy about beta-carotene as a supplement, there is no disagreement about the powerful qualities of this substance found in natural foods and its ability to keep you younger. When you get it by eating fruits and vegetables, you get all the forms of the substance that nature intends you to get so your body can enjoy its youth-enhancing properties.

Get your share of such naturally sweet foods as sweet potatoes, carrots, pumpkin, spinach, and you'll get enough beta-carotene to get more powerful NK cells and an immune system with twice the power.

The ability of this power food to keep you younger is even more important as you reach maturity, when the immune system starts to decline with the years. A mere 60 mg. of beta-carotene daily results in a significant increase in the percentage of NK cells and T-cells.

### Power Food V: Foods Containing the Minerals Copper and Zinc

Both copper and zinc help keep the immune system operating at full efficiency, building strong defenses through T-cells and antibodies.

Once you reach middle age, the thymus gland begins to shrink and reduce its output of thymulin. This reduction becomes significantly marked after age 60. Daily low doses of zinc can result in as much as 80 percent regrowth of the thymus gland with significant increases in the number of T-cells. When 15 mg. of zinc per day were supplied to a group of individuals over the age of 65, their T-cell activity was as efficient as that of much younger people.

Power foods that contain copper are dried peas and beans, fruits and shellfish. Those containing zinc are cereals, beans, turkey and oysters.

All these power foods contain building blocks that keep the immune system from aging, thereby helping to maintain a healthier, more attractive body ten more years.

# YOUTH-BUILDING VITAMINS AND MINERALS

Vitamin and mineral supplements can help us live longer. We're better off getting these substances directly from food sources, but most of us can't count on eating enough of and the right amounts of such foods all the time. So supplements are an insurance policy that, just in case we're not getting all our vitamins directly from the food sources, we're sure to get them in supplement form. As such they're relatively inexpensive, relatively safe from side effects and a form of health maintenance that we can control easily. Supplements are one of the tickets to ride to ten more years of healthy, attractive living.

Taking the regimen of vitamins and minerals recommended in this chapter will help you live ten years longer, live more comfortably and look more attractive by helping to:

1.  Avoid the onset of various types of cancers.

2.  Decrease the risk of heart and circulatory diseases.

3.  Lower cholesterol levels.

4.  Improve circulation.

5.  Slow down the aging process through antioxidants.

6.  Promote the effective functioning of your immune system.

7.  Protect against environmental pollution and food additives.

8.  Fight viral infections.

9.  Prevent anemia.

10. Detoxify harmful substances.

11. Get rid of poisonous metals such as mercury and cadmium.

12. Alleviate symptoms and disabilities of rheumatoid arthritis.

13. Reduce your craving for sweets, thereby helping you to lose weight (see section on chromium picolinate).

14. Keep your skin healthy.

## Vitamins Prolong Life

Naturally occurring substances in your diet can help prevent the "rusting" or aging process. The most common of these elements are the vitamins C, E, and beta-carotene, and minerals such as selenium and zinc. Although these substances do occur naturally in our diets, they may not be in sufficient quantity to prolong our lives as much as we'd like.

# VITAMIN C: LINUS PAULING'S PROMISE OF YOUTH

Dr. Linus Pauling had clearly spent more time researching the benefits of vitamin C than any other human being on this planet. He was unequivocally a strong advocate of its benefits and had written a good deal to substantiate his claims. Although the conventional regimen for vitamin C recommended by nutritionists is about 60 mg. per day, Pauling himself ingested 18 grams (18,000 mg.) each and every day of his adult life. But Dr. Pauling didn't recommend that for everyone.

Pauling stressed very strongly that each individual has a unique biochemistry that calls for different amounts of vitamin C, ranging from as little as one quarter of a gram a day to 20 or more grams per day. So how do you discover your own optimal regimen?

First of all, you must begin by realizing that vitamin C is one of the very few substances that cannot seriously harm you through overdosing. Research has shown that even an equivalent of 350 grams (350,000 mg.) a day will not be very harmful. What does happen is that when you reach your optimal dosage, anything beyond that will cause diarrhea. That's nature's subtle way of telling you when you've reached your optimal dosage. When you reach that point, you merely scale back a bit until you regain normalcy once again. Vitamin C is virtually nontoxic. But more specifically, what can vitamin C, at optimal dosage, do to help extend your lifespan?

## How Vitamin C Adds Years to Life

Since colds rarely kill us, how can vitamin C extend our lifespan? The answer to that is in the fact that vitamin C plays a much more major role in our bodies than that of resisting colds. Thousands and thousands of published scientific papers all point to the pervasive effect of vitamin C on all the physiological processes going on within our bodies. For a brief summary, vitamin C:

1. plays a very important role in the health of our heart and its entire vascular system;

2. can play a very important role in the prevention and treatment of cancer;

3. promotes the healing of tissue wounds;

4. aids in the prevention of broken bones;

5. plays a very significant role in keeping our immune systems functioning in a healthy manner;

6. helps overcome male infertility;

7. counteracts the symptoms of asthma;

8. protects against smoking and various pollutants;

9. helps prevent diabetes, in terms of sugar and energy metabolism.

### Thirty-five More Years

This is not to say that vitamin C alone will extend your life span. Obviously, woman does not live by C alone. Other vitamins and minerals as well as healthier lifestyle habits in general are necessary to live longer, more youthful lives. If we take charge of our diets and other habits, then we have a comprehensive grasp on controlling the length and quality of our lives. "My estimate, made on the basis of the results of epidemiological and other observations," said Dr. Pauling, "is that through the optimum use of vitamin supplements and other health measures, the length of the period of well-being and the length of life could be increased by twenty-five to thirty-five years."

### At Least Ten More Years

I'm a bit more modest. I'm just promising you ten more years of youthful, enjoyable life. I'd rather be conservative in what I hope for. But that's ten more years than you would otherwise have.

What are the more important functions of the vitamins, in addition to what we've already discussed? Here are some answers, in alphabetical order.

### Vitamin A Purifies the Blood

The chief function of vitamin A, stored in the liver, is the purification of the blood from such pollutants as pesticides, industrial poisons, and the toxic side effects of prescribed medications. It sometimes also retards the development of cancerous tumors of the breast and cervix. However, it is preferable to take beta-carotene, which is converted to vitamin A by the body as needed, and thereby prevents the possibility of overdosing on this fat-soluble vitamin.

## Choose Niacin over Niacinamide

The reason I recommend the niacin form of B3 (which causes flush-
ing) over the niacinamide form (which doesn't) is because only
niacin has been found to reduce cholesterol and triglyceride levels,
perhaps even reversing atherosclerosis. Scientists researching this
function of niacin claim that no other single agent has such potential for lowering both cholesterol and triglycerides. Taking niacin
after meals (as you should all vitamin pills) should reduce the flush-
ing.

Vitamin $B_6$ is one of the most important B vitamins. It:

1. protects against cancer,

2. helps keep the skin healthy, and

3. boosts the immune system.

Pantothenic acid is useful not only in alleviating the painful
symptoms and disability of rheumatoid arthritis but also in extending the lifespan by 18 to 20 percent. I recommend a dosage of 30
mg./day.

Vitamin C has already been discussed in depth.

Vitamin D is produced naturally on the skin of the body in the
presence of sunlight and absorbed into the body. Only if you are
deprived of sunlight do you need to worry about sufficient levels of
this. A lack of it will make you more vulnerable to breast cancer.

Vitamin E has been mentioned in its function as an aid in heart-
related problems. It has also been known, in conjunction with selenium, to slow the growth of cancer cells in blood plasma. Vitamin E
is able to dissolve blood clots in the circulatory system. It also
improves circulation, as well as protects us against some environmental toxins. By its action on free radicals, vitamin E can extend the
lifespan.

## The Power of Minerals

The essential difference between vitamins and minerals is that vitamins are organic (bound chemically to carbon), whereas minerals are
not, except for the trace minerals selenium and chromium. Minerals
necessary for good health include compounds of the basic elements
calcium, chlorine, magnesium, phosphorus, potassium, and sulfur.

Also, trace elements of the following minerals are essential: chromium, copper, iodine, iron, manganese, molybdenum, and zinc.

### COPPER PROTECTS MEMBRANES AND RELIEVES ARTHRITIS. *Copper* is an important antioxidant, which inhibits free-radical formation from reduced iron, and maintains the integrity of cell membranes. It is an important defense in lung membranes for chronic smokers.

Copper bracelets have long been thought to help battle the painful symptoms of arthritis. As the copper is absorbed through sweat and skin into the body and subsequently into the synovial fluid of the affected joints, the sufferers of osteoarthritis as well as rheumatoid arthritis can expect some relief.

### MAGNESIUM FOR HEART AND BLOOD PRESSURE. *Magnesium* is very important for healthy cardiac function. It is essential to the electrical and physical integrity of the heart. It also helps control blood pressure, as well as curb free radicals and keep bones strong.

### MANGANESE—PREVENTS DEGENERATIVE PROCESS. *Manganese*, another antioxidant, is so important to human biology that nature has provided for it to be substituted by magnesium in many biochemical reactions when deficiencies occur. What role does manganese play in extending your life for ten years? Well, according to the latest research, all tumors have diminished amounts of the manganese-containing enzyme. Manganese deficiency may play a role in degenerative processes in humans.

Although manganese is considered safe up to 10 mg./day, I recommend a 2–5 mg./day dose, since it is available in fruits, green vegetables, and whole grains, all of which I recommend highly.

### ZINC KEEPS IMMUNE SYSTEM YOUNG. Research has shown that as we age we become increasingly prone to *zinc* deficiency. Yet more than one hundred enzymes require the trace metal zinc, including the production of DNA and RNA, as well as cell membranes. Zinc is believed to maintain membrane cell integrity.

The older we get, the less efficient our immune system. If we also get less zinc in our maturing years, we may be at risk. Progressive zinc deficiency may have something to do with our aging immune system. For instance, in the laboratory, zinc-deficient animals show much greater susceptibility to cancer caused by chemicals. A certain breed of cattle (Dutch Friesian - A46 mutant) cannot absorb zinc from their feed, making them extremely susceptible to infection and early death. The cure for this terrible disease? Their lifespan is significantly increased by the supplementation of zinc.

There is some evidence that zinc may help those suffering from chronic rheumatoid arthritis by reducing swelling and stiffness. Since our ability to absorb zinc diminishes with age, high-fiber diets result in lower zinc absorption, and excessive sweating due to exercise causes a loss of existing zinc, zinc supplementation is essential. Fortunately, most multivitamin pills contain at least 15 mg. of zinc. And that's the amount I recommend.

CHROMIUM PICOLINATE HELPS REDUCE CRAVINGS FOR SWEETS AND MAY AID IN WEIGHT LOSS. Chromium is best known for its function in supporting insulin's role in sugar metabolism. The trivalent form of chromium in the form of a substance called glucose tolerance factor is found in *brewer's yeast*. A deficiency in chromium results in higher cholesterol levels, cholesterol deposits in the arteries, and a shorter lifespan, as well as glucose intolerance. Unfortunately, as we age, we can expect dramatic declines in the concentration of this important element in our bloodstream.

Of all the vitamins and minerals, chromium is more likely to be in short supply than any other substance in the American diet. Ninety percent of us consume less than 50 micrograms daily, even though the amount recommended by the National Academy of Science is 50 to 200 mcg. daily.

It is important to distinguish between the two types of chromium. *Trivalent* or *nutritional chromium* is the good type and has very low toxicity; *hexavalent chromium* is highly toxic, leading to skin problems and lung cancer. But there's no need to worry as far as supplements are concerned. The bad chromium would come in the form of environmental pollution. The good chromium, in the form of chromium trichloride or *chromium picolinate*, known as biologically active chromium, is what we find in food and supplements.

There is some intriguing evidence that chromium picolinate effectively reduces the craving for sweets and helps some people lose more fat than those on similar diets without chromium. Perhaps it is precisely because American women may be suffering from chromium deficiency that makes them so susceptible to processed sweet foods.

MOLYBDENUM—DETOXIFIES HARMFUL SUBSTANCES. *Molybdenum's* function is to detoxify potentially harmful substances we come across daily. Although I recommend 50 micrograms per day, the amount you get in most vitamin pills (up to 25 mcg.) should be adequate. Although this substance plays an important antioxidant role, this role is very complex, and molybdenum in the soil giving rise to the foods we eat is at least as important as its supplementary form.

SELENIUM ANTICANCER, ANTIHEART DISEASE, PROIMMUNE SYSTEM. And finally, the superstar of trace elements: *selenium*. It used to be considered a potential carcinogen. Now it's hailed as a protection *against* cancer and a number of other diseases, as well as contributing to the extension of life. Selenium serves as an antioxidant that prevents damage to cellular membranes.

Another very important quality is that selenium aids in the prevention of cancer. A growing number of studies reveals that the lower the levels of selenium in the food and water, the higher the incidence of various forms of cancer. This is true in comparing various regions of the U.S. as well as comparing various countries. Japan, for example, has a higher selenium level than the U.S.; so Japanese individuals have a smaller incidence of cancer—until they emigrate to the U.S. Other research has revealed higher levels of selenium in the blood of healthy individuals than in those suffering from cancer.

Research also points to selenium as a significant boost to the immune system. Animal studies reveal that selenium supplements, when accompanied by vitamin E, lead to large increases in antibody production, as well as improved lymphocytic activity.

Selenium also acts to protect the heart and circulatory system. Research comparing different regions and countries reveals a striking relationship between selenium levels and heart disease. The lower the selenium soil content, the greater the number of deaths from heart disease. Selenium, along with vitamin E, appears to prevent free-radical damage to the blood vessels in the heart.

Selenium can also "police" other poisonous metals such as mercury and cadmium. It is hypothesized that it does so by combining with these metals to form inert, harmless selenides—in effect "handcuffing" itself to these "criminal" metals to take them out of circulation.

So for all these benefits, 200 micrograms per day is recommended. In addition to your multivitamin pill, at least consider an additional combination pill of selenium and vitamin E if you're too busy to coordinate a precise regimen.

## The Basics: Daily Multivitamin + C

A respectable multiple vitamin is the base from which to start. If nothing else, at least take this multiple vitamin once a day with 500 to 1,000 mg. tablets of vitamin C as often as you need to get your optimal dosage of vitamin C. Spread the vitamin C dosage throughout the day as much as possible. Remember, this vitamin is water soluble and is not stored in the body. In addition, you might consider a B-complex tablet.

Vitamins do not work as well in isolation as they do in concert. This is especially true of the B vitamins. So a B-complex tablet is worth considering as part of your vitamin regimen.

# SOME CAUTIONS ABOUT VITAMINS

## Avoid Time-release Niacin

Vitamin B3 (the niacin form) causes some people to feel a tingly flush over their skin. This is a normal reaction and the best way to deal with it is to see it as insurance that the vitamin is working. Niacin serves to reduce blood cholesterol levels when taken in dosages of at least 500 mg. per day. However, at levels of over 2,000 mg. a day, medical supervision should be obtained because in some very few cases temporary side effects that affect the liver have been documented. This problem has been noticed primarily with time-release forms of niacin and in higher dosages.

## Take Your Vitamins After Meals

Two cautions for vitamin C. This vitamin is somewhat acid and may cause stomach distress when taken in high dosages, so it is best to take this (and all other vitamins) after meals. Another way to deal with this problem if it exists is to take the vitamin in the form of sodium ascorbate. The second note of caution is exclusively for diabetics taking medicinal insulin. Since vitamin C increases the efficiency of insulin, it can disrupt the delicate sugar-insulin balance in diabetics. In such a case, it would be wise to have medical supervision when beginning a regimen of vitamin C.

### High Blood Pressure? Consult Your Doctor

Medical supervision is also advised for those who have high blood pressure (150/90 or higher) and are taking more than 100 IU of vitamin E. Remember that this vitamin strengthens the heart muscle.

### Divide Your Vitamin C Dosages Throughout the Day

If at all possible, it is best to divide your dosages throughout the day. Do this as much as possible, especially with vitamin C. It is well known that C does not build up in the bloodstream. So taking it on an hourly basis would be best. The next best would be after every meal and snack, and so on.

## SOME CAUTIONS ABOUT MINERALS

It is important to beware of certain circumstances that would be exceptions to the rule of the mineral regimen recommended.

For example, for anyone with preexisting high calcium concentrations in the blood, any calcium supplementation beyond a daily multivitamin should be avoided. Copper supplements should be avoided by those suffering from *hepatolenticular degeneration* (Wilson's disease); women with renal failure should avoid magnesium; and anyone with high uric acid levels or suffering from gout should avoid molybdenum. Finally, selenium in dosages of 200 mcg. per day is considered to be entirely safe, but at high dosages (1,000 mcg. per day) it can become problematic. So be mindful of the dosages of all your supplements, but especially selenium.

## A Word of Reassurance

Having offered you cautionary advice about nutritional supplements, I now want to ease your mind that, given the conservatively moderate doses in the regimen I recommend, you are quite safe. I want to end this section on nutritional supplements with the words of Dr. Bernard Rimland, a leading theorist on nutritional therapy, who claims that:

> *Vitamins are extraordinarily nontoxic.* The only vitamins that are remotely toxic are vitamins A and D, and the toxicity of vitamin A is greatly exaggerated. I think that there has been only one person in 12 years who has died of vitamin A overdose. He had to consume millions and millions of units of vitamin A.

So, as you make use of nutritional supplements to ensure the primary component of our program to add ten youthful years to your life, rest assured that what you are doing is based on years of conventional scientific research and well within the margins of safety as determined by our scientific and medical communities.

## SUPERFOODS FOR INCREASED BRAIN POWER

*Nootropics* is the name given to drugs that make the brain work better. My own research indicates that much of this lore is full of hype and exaggeration. Here is the bottom line on what works and what doesn't.

## What Doesn't Work

Two of the most highly touted "smart" drugs are *deprenyl* and *piracetam*. Deprenyl, which helps the brain release the neurotransmitter *dopamine*, has proven successful in helping those suffering from Alzheimer's and Parkinson's diseases. By inference, it also may assist the normal brain in working more efficiently. However, what works for the diseased brain does not necessarily help the normal brain.

Piracetam has proven successful in a few studies. In one study it is reported to have improved the alertness and aptitude of elderly drivers. In another study of 18 elderly people, it showed "marked gains in mental performance." But much more conclusive research is needed before I'd recommend such drugs. Let's take a look at what clearly does work.

### How to B Smart

Three B vitamins—$B_6$, $B_{12}$, and folic acid—are necessary for the brain to produce the neurotransmitters serotonin and norepinephrine, which control alertness. A respectable body of evidence reveals that too little of these vitamins may result in mental sluggishness and even depression.

As we get older, we tend to produce lower levels of these vitamins. Many women over 65 have low levels of at least one of these three vitamins. Among such mature individuals, those with the lowest levels of $B_{12}$ and folic acid scored the worst on tests of memory and reasoning in a study of over 250 subjects. Correcting this deficiency proves successful in improving concentration and memory. Having adequate amounts of these B vitamins seems to part the clouds of foggy thinking.

### Feeling Stressed? Can't Concentrate? Try Tyrosine!

*Tyrosine* is an amino acid which is converted by the brain to *norepinephrine*, one of the neurotransmitters mentioned previously. This substance can be depleted when we're under stress for prolonged periods. Tyrosine pills have proven effective in helping women under stress to concentrate more effectively.

### The Afternoon Slump

There are two reasons for the common afternoon slump. One has to do with time, the other with food. There seems to be a natural cycle of decreasing arousal that occurs around midafternoon, affecting some individuals more than others. Some European and Mediterranean cultures even close down their commerce for a midafternoon siesta and then open up shop again about 4 P.M. American women work right through it, or at least try to.

The other reason, food, has to do with the amount and type of food we consume for lunch. A lunch made up predominantly of carbohydrates, such as starchy and sweet foods, stimulates the release of insulin, which lowers the level of most amino acids but not tryptophan. The result? A drowsy midafternoon slump. On the other hand, a lunch made up primarily of proteins causes the tryptophan to be bullied aside by the other amino acids, resulting in an alert mind that is able to concentrate well.

The size of the lunch matters as well. A large lunch will result in much more drowsiness than a small lunch. So the best option for an alert, effective brain and for a most productive afternoon is a rather small lunch made up of more protein than carbohydrates.

# REDUCING YOUR RISK OF CANCER

The amazing thing about preventing cancer through nutrition is the simplicity of it all. Just imagine a preindustrialized farmer who has never eaten the meat of an animal or any of its products (milk, eggs), and that diet is the perfect anticancer regimen.

## Low Fat, High Fiber

The National Cancer Institute (NCI) recommends a lot of dietary fiber: breads made with whole grains, fruits, vegetables, and beans. It urges the reduction of fat, which comes primarily from meat, fowl, and dairy products. That's exactly how our preindustrial farmer eats. No sophisticated diets or supplements are needed.

## How to Eat to Prevent Cancer

Our lives aren't as simple. So here are some suggestions to reduce your risk of cancer.

1. Help yourself to a serving of whole-grain bread, cereal, pasta, or brown rice at least four times a day. That is, have at least six

servings of any of this variety of foods at least four times a day, in any combination.

2. Have at least two (1-oz.) servings each day of citrus fruits, green peppers, or tomatoes.

3. At least once a day, help yourself to some broccoli, cabbage, carrots, or cauliflower.

4. Enjoy some beans or peas a few times a week.

5. If you're not a vegetarian, choose fish or fowl (white meat) over red meat. If you must have your meat, be sure it's trimmed of fat.

**What *not* to eat:**

6. Avoid whole-milk dairy products such as whole milk itself, ice cream and high-fat cheeses. If you must have cheese, choose 2 percent cottage or skim milk mozzarella.

7. Avoid fried foods if you know what's good for you, because butter, margarine, and shortening, aren't. This includes sour cream, oil, and so on. Air-popped popcorn is great—just say "No butter, please."

8. Never eat hot dogs, sausage, or processed luncheon meats.

## Stay Within Ten Pounds of Your Ideal Weight

If you can do all this and stay within 10 pounds of your ideal weight, then you've got a good head start in keeping cancer from stealing any of those ten precious years you're earning.

## The Skinny on Fat

Now for some commentary. First, on fat: As you're probably aware, there are three kinds of fat. *Saturated fats* are usually found in red meat, poultry skin, and fried foods. *Monounsaturated fats* are found primarily in peanuts and olives. *Polyunsaturated fats* are found in corn, safflower, and other cooking oils. To overcome the dietary complexity of it all, a good anticancer regimen would decrease saturated fats (meat and fried foods) and allow a bit more of the other two types.

## How Fat Causes Cancer

It is not clear exactly how fat contributes to cancer formation. One theory holds that fat upsets the body's hormone balance and increases hormone levels of estrogen, androgen and prolactin. Another theory maintains that bile acids, produced by the body to break down fats, create by-products which help promote the development of cancer. Whichever theory proves correct, the result is a greater vulnerability to cancer.

## Whole Milk vs. Skim Milk

Here's some proof. One study of over 4,600 individuals examined the participants' milk-drinking habits. It found that those who drank skim milk or 2 percent milk had a significantly lower risk of cancer than those who drank whole milk. Remember that 2 percent milk has twice as much fat as 1 percent milk, and whole milk has twice as much fat as 2 percent milk.

But intriguingly, it was discovered that those who drank no milk at all had more cancer than those who drank skim milk. So milk is good for you (probably because of its vitamins and calcium), but only if you drink the skim variety with the lowest proportion of fat. So a very important move is to shift from whole milk to 2 percent milk for a few weeks to get used to it. Then gradually shift to skim milk.

In another large-scale study, this one of over 10,000 women worldwide, Dr. Geoffrey Howe found a consistent correlation between higher intake of saturated fat and higher breast-cancer risk for postmenopausal women. He also found a relationship between higher dietary vitamin C and lower risk of cancer.

## How Fiber Helps Prevent Cancer

One more large-scale study involving over 10,000 people revealed that diets low in fat and high in vegetables and other high-fiber foods were related to a significantly lower incidence of colon cancer. That's why I stress eating so many servings of whole grain breads and cereals. You need to replace the fats with more fiber. The fiber not only replaces the fat; it also speeds up the movement of food in the intestines as well, and dilutes potential carcinogens.

## Peel or Wash Your Produce

Most of us are used to consuming only 10 to 12 grams of fiber a day. To help prevent cancer, we need more like 25 to 30 grams each day. In addition to carbohydrates, don't forget fruits and vegetables—pears, apples, bananas, and beans. A wide variety works much better than focusing on any one source of fiber. This also helps prevent exposure to any one type of carcinogen that might be present in pesticides. It also helps to wash produce well before eating or cooking. And when possible, it is advisable to peel fruits and vegetables for the same reason, even though this means losing some of the nutrients.

## Why Hot Dogs Are Bad for You

One of my suggestions earlier in this chapter was to avoid hot dogs and sausages. Here's why: Hot dogs and most processed meats contain *sodium nitrite* and *sodium nitrate* both as a preservative and as a color and flavor enhancer. Nitrate by itself is harmless. But it is easily converted into the other type of nitrite, which is not. Nitrite combines with compounds called *secondary amines* to produce highly carcinogenic *nitrosamines*, either during the cooking process or during digestion. Food processors have been forced by the government to reduce nitrite levels in past years, but it is still there, albeit not as much as it used to be. So avoid hot dogs. Opt for air-popped popcorn (without butter) at the movies.

## Why Some Produce Is Waxed

Since I'm promoting fruit so highly, I need to mention this cautionary note. Many fruits and vegetables are waxed, both to prevent moisture loss and to enhance visual appeal. It is virtually impossible to know which produce has been waxed (except in such obvious cases as apples and cucumbers).

## Why You Should Peel or Wash

Here's the problem. Fungicides are frequently applied before waxing, or mixed with the wax solution. Some of the FDA-approved fungicides, such as *benomyl*, *captan*, and *folpet* are associated with increased risk of cancer. Although this is most probably not a significant risk because of the minute amounts per serving, it is a good idea to peel whenever possible, wash whenever you can, and if you're able, avoid buying produce from Chile and Mexico, where higher pesticide residues are allowed.

## Effects of Diet on Breast Cancer

Later on, I'll be suggesting a Food Plan which should bring you close to reducing your fat intake to 20 percent of total calories. According to research, breast cancer has the closest link to dietary fat of all cancers. To further decrease your chances of breast cancer, make sure to increase your fiber intake to 25 or more grams per day. Cutting your fat intake will decrease tumor-stimulating fatty acids and estrogen blood levels.

Eating more fruits and vegetables will not only provide more fiber, but will also provide more beta carotene, which will help keep you cancer-free.

## Effects of Diet on Cancer of the Cervix

Although there are many causes of cervical cancer—nutritional deficits, and sexual history, for example—the number of deaths due to cervical cancer has decreased by about 50 percent in the last few decades, thanks in great part to detection by the Pap smear.

The best dietary approach to fight cervical cancer, especially if you have a family history of this, is a combination of antioxidant supplements such as vitamin C and beta carotene, as well as folic acid.

## Effects of Diet on Colon Cancer

Again, the best approach to prevention is a low-fat, high-fiber diet. In addition to that, research suggests adding foods rich in beta-carotene; allium vegetables, such as garlic, onion and leeks; plus calcium supplements.

The fiber helps to rush the carcinogens in food through the lower bowel more quickly. Fat may increase the production of bile acids which can promote tumors on the colon wall. Calcium can counteract the harmful effects of the bile acids. The sulfur chemicals in allium vegetables can actually inhibit cancer growth. So there's a definite reason for all these anticolon cancer components.

# DR. RYBACK'S ANTIAGING WEIGHT LOSS PROGRAM

There are two phases to losing weight. The first is a more or less sudden dramatic shift in your eating habits; the second is a maintenance phase which ideally lasts a lifetime. There is no doubt about the importance of the first phase. It helps establish a sense of control and mastery over your body. Most quick diets accomplish this by producing a rapid loss of water in the body, which will result in a psychologically satisfying loss of weight in very short order. As long as weight is dramatically reduced in the short term, all appears well on the surface.

The same effect can be achieved, if you are determined to experience the psychological boost, by making a decision about some aspects of your eating habits. There is no replacement for the decrease in food intake, so one way to go about losing weight quickly is to cut your food intake drastically. Fasting is the most dramatic way to do it, but probably not the most sensible for most people. Nevertheless, some may find it effective as a starting point. So if you do consider this option, do so carefully.

## How to Make Hunger Pangs Work for You

Your first concern might be that feeling of hunger that comes from the pit of your stomach. I have learned to translate that feeling as a signal that says to me that this is what it feels like to be in the process of becoming thinner. Whether you call it a process of meditation, self-hypnosis, or rationalization, the net result is that what could be considered painful and uncomfortable is suddenly transformed into a sensation of victory over obesity and mastery over one's own body. To the extent that I can really feel my hunger pangs as positive feedback to my own body, I am already being rewarded for my decrease in eating. There is no need to weigh myself in order to get this successful feedback. Eventually the "hunger pangs" become a signal for success and an instant source of self-esteem.

This process of transforming "hunger pangs" into positive feedback will certainly take some investment of time and energy on your part. You can begin taking 10 to 20 minutes before breakfast or before you leave home in the morning to sit in a calm, quiet spot and meditate on this process. You can either repeat to yourself silently the affirmation, "This empty sensation makes me feel thinner and successful in mastery over my own body," or merely meditate upon the process in a style that is comfortable for you.

## Taking Charge

You may argue that hunger pangs are nature's way of telling you that your body needs food and that these signals should be obeyed. If you feel that way and you are as thin as you'd like to be, then you're absolutely right. However, if you are overweight, then obviously your body has been fibbing and excess weight is the unhappy result. So the choice is ultimately yours. If you are happy with your body weight, listen to the body signals to eat when you feel hunger. If, on the other hand, you want to become thinner, then you need to teach yourself to interpret your body signals in a new way. If you truly want to become thinner, then you can do so by making a conscious, intelligent decision about when you will and will not eat rather than let your body signals make the decision for you. Having transformed the interpretation of your body signals, you are now in charge. From this vantage point, you can now decide to what degree of "suddenness" you want to become thinner.

Incidentally, one ballpark way of figuring your ideal weight is to start at 100 pounds for five feet, and then add five pounds for each additional inch, plus or minus 10 pounds.

## Lose No More than 2 Pounds a Week

Eating is a very complex activity. Each culture has its own customs and traditions with regard to eating. Each person has his or her own eating habits as well. In our culture, more specifically in the advertising aspects, of our culture, we can be seduced with promises of losing 10 to 20 pounds in a single week. Whether women actually accomplish this or not, I'd consider it quite unhealthy. A much healthier and more moderate approach, in my opinion, is to consider losing a pound or two a week at the most. Anything more sudden than that would be unhealthy. Having said this, let me now offer some specific options for you to consider.

### The Fasting Option

At the most extreme, you may consider the fasting option just mentioned. Fasting every other day is an option that will drastically decrease your food intake in an obvious way. Even if you eat as much food as you have always eaten on the days that you do eat, choosing this option will certainly have a dramatic impact on your weight. Some women become lightheaded and somewhat uncomfortable, even dizzy, when they try this. If you are such an individual, then this option is not for you. So let's move on to less dramatic possibilities.

### The Option of Fewer Meals

The next option consists of eating only one or two meals a day rather than the usual three. If you choose this option, give considerable thought to what feels right for you. Some women feel comfortable waiting until dinner time so that they can reward themselves at the end of a day in which they did not eat. Others, on the other hand, may feel they need a considerable-sized breakfast, some lunch, and then not eat anything for the rest of the day except for a light snack in the evening. Another option is to have no breakfast and an early lunch and call it brunch, thereby condensing two meals into one.

### The Most Highly Recommended Option

The healthiest option and the one I strongly recommend is to have a light breakfast, a morning snack, a light lunch, a midafternoon snack, and look forward to dinner as the main meal of the day. The important thing to remember is that each time you eat, keep it light.

## BE THIN WITHOUT BEING HUNGRY

Here is a sample food plan which will keep you eating throughout the day and allow you to lose weight in the process. This is the food plan

I highly recommend, in terms of minimal deprivation, nutritional sensibility, and metabolic efficiency. It's a five-course food plan that I strongly encourage.

## THE RYBACK FOOD PLAN

**Breakfast**

 Fruit (grapefruit, orange) either whole or as juice
 High-fiber cereal with skim milk, topped occasionally with fruit
 Whole-wheat toast or bagel (with apple butter or jelly)

**10:00 A.M.**

 Small apple, peach, or $1/4$ cup of raisins, or English muffin

**Lunch**

 Baked potato, brown rice, or pasta with small bits of fish or poultry
 Green vegetable or 1 large carrot
 Mineral water, fruit juice, or skim milk
      *or*
 Bowl of your favorite homemade vegetable soup
 Green salad with oil-free dressing
 Whole wheat roll
 Fruit cup or 1 apple

**3:00 P.M.**

 A fruit such as apple, peach, banana, raisins or nonfat yogurt

**Dinner**

 Start with mineral water and fruit cocktail
 2–3 ounces of broiled flounder, sole or skinless chicken
  (white meat) or turkey breast
 2 vegetables or green salad
 Baked potato, pasta, or brown rice with shiitake mushrooms
 Dessert of two fruits blended

The Ryback Food Plan allows for fruit or fruit juice 5 times a day and allows for a vegetable serving at both lunch and dinner. Whole-wheat bread or rolls can be eaten at any of the meals. A choice of pasta, rice, or a baked potato (without fattening condiments) is allowed for both lunch and dinner. High-protein foods such as fish or skinless fowl are recommended for the dinner meal, although there's no reason not to eat such food at lunch instead if that meal is traditionally the larger one for you.

I recommend you get in the habit of eating your protein food as an adornment to a rice or pasta dish rather than by itself. You really don't need a lot of high-protein food and if you get in the habit of eating it to add flavor to your rice or pasta dish, you'll enjoy it at least as much and you'll be getting into healthier eating habits.

If you stick to the Ryback Food Plan, you won't have to worry about singling out foods that make you fat, such as fried foods, cake and cookies, candy and chocolates, creams and sauces, high-fat dairy and beef products. Nor do you have to count calories. By flavoring your rice or pasta dishes with different high-protein foods and vegetables, you have an infinite variety of dishes you can look forward to. If you do choose to use sauces, make sure they're as fat-free as possible. Rather than focus on dietary restrictions, the Ryback Food Plan focuses on what's good for you and allows you the choice to be as creative as you would like with healthy foods.

As you read through Chapter Nine on building a strong heart, you'll notice that this same food plan works for that purpose as well. The Ryback Food Plan not only keeps you thin, it will also lower your cholesterol levels, and is very similar to what is recommended as a cancer-prevention diet.

For those of you who cannot bear the thought of giving up all those foods that are bad for you but seduce your taste buds, you can solve the problem by going on a food orgy one meal a week or, better yet, one meal a month. On that food "holiday" you can eat as much as you want of whatever you want, as long as you restrict it to that one time a week or month. What's really important is what happens over the long run. As long as the "orgy" meals happen only once in a while, and that helps you stay healthy the rest of the time, then its okay. You deserve the holiday if you're eating healthfully the rest of the time. This isn't about deprivation—it's about helping you live ten years longer!

## MINIMIZING THE DISCOMFORTS OF PMS

*Premenstrual syndrome* affects one third to one half of all American women between 20 and 50. It is, unfortunately, the target of many jokes, but to women who suffer from the physical, emotional, and behavioral symptoms, it's not funny at all.

PMS has been classified into four different types:

1. *Type* A includes anxiety, irritability, and mood swings.

2. *Type* B involves sugar craving, headaches, and fatigue.

3. *Type* H stands for hyperhydration. This means bloating, weight gain, and breast tenderness.

4. *Type* D involves depression, confusion, memory loss, and occasionally, violent behavior.

And there are other symptoms, too, including acne, asthma, hoarseness, backache, painful knees and ankles, dizziness, fainting, and alcoholic binges. Whatever symptoms you have, be they mild or severe, seven to ten days before your period they will occur, much to your dismay.

Women who don't exercise, have trouble maintaining their weight, and lead high-stress lives seem to be at a higher risk for PMS. Poor eating habits such as consuming junk food, red meat, caffeine, and sugar, or going for long periods without eating anything, also seem to trigger ths syndrome.

### What Causes PMS?

There are multiple causes for PMS, and although several have been clearly identified, there hasn't been much research and results haven't always been conclusive. There are a few different threads within this fabric—hormonal, biochemical, neuroendocrinal, psychological, and psychosocial. Some possible causes are:

1. *Low beta-endorphin activity during the luteal phase* (second half of the menstrual cycle). Here, the brain isn't properly producing those natural opiates that alleviate pain and make you feel good, so you may suffer from mood swings.

2. *Serotonin deficiency.* This neurotransmitter is responsible for your sense of well-being, and during the last 10 days of the cycle of women with PMS, there are lower blood serotonin levels.

3. *Progesterone withdrawal.* Progesterone levels decrease just before your period, and women with PMS have less of this hormone just as their symptoms are getting worse.

4. *High prolactin levels.* Breast tenderness may be caused by an increase of this pituitary hormone in the brain which is secreted during breastfeeding but is also present in nonlactating women.

Other causes appear to be *abnormal prostaglandin metabolism, hypoglycemia* (reduced blood sugar), and *hypothyroidism* (low thyroid function). Others believe that it may also be a sleep disorder, since the hormones that make you sleepy at appropriate times drop at ovulation. For some women, feeling exhausted can lead to other symptoms.

## How to Minimize the Symptoms of PMS

1. *Eat regularly and often.* In order to stabilize this condition, you need to eat differently during this time of the month. Since your mechanism for controlling blood sugar is off, it's advisable to have a high-carbohydrate snack every three hours or so, to keep blood sugar on an even keel. A slice of bread, some cereal, a potato, or a serving of rice will do the trick. Don't allow yourself to get hungry—carry crackers or a bagel with you if you're going to be out and about for any long period.

2. *Consume enough liquid.* Drink eight glasses of water a day, especially one week before and one week after your period.

3. *Increase calcium.* You can follow my Osteoporosis-Prevention Diet in Chapter 7. More calcium during the premenstrual period has been found to reduce mood, concentration, and behavior problems and reduce water retention.

4. *Stop smoking; stop drinking caffeine.* Both cigarettes and caffeinated products make symptoms worse.

5. *Reduce stress and get enough sleep.* A good daily program of tai chi chuan, yoga, or meditation is valuable in reducing PMS symptoms.

And if you get enough sleep—7 to 8 hours a night—you will undoubtedly feel refreshed enough to continue throughout the day. Some women with PMS suffer from *seasonal affective disorder* (see Chapter Four, p. 105) and may benefit from light therapy.

# SPECIAL NUTRITIONAL NEEDS OF THE PREGNANT WOMAN

The entire body changes physically, chemically, and mechanically during pregnancy. The blood volume is nearly doubled, and blood pressure typically rises as do blood sugar levels. And of course, there are dozens of possible discomforts typical to pregnancy that might affect your gastrointestinal system, including heartburn, nausea, bloating and constipation.

## Weight Gain

The average woman gains from 15 to 40 pounds over the course of her pregnancy, depending on what she weighs before conception, her fitness level, body type, and eating habits. Half of this weight gain can be attributed to the fetus, placenta, and amniotic fluid; the other half, the part that's called "maternal stores," is quite literally stored just in case anything should happen to the mother's food supply and starvation might threaten to endanger the baby within. To a certain degree, water retention also makes you heavier than you might otherwise be.

Thinner women need to gain more weight to support a pregnancy; heavier women already have good fat stores and should watch their diet to be sure that they're only ingesting "full" rather than "empty" calories.

## A Good Diet

When you're pregnant, you need the best diet available with an additional helping of calcium for the good bone growth of your fetus. If you follow my Osteoporosis Prevention Diet in Chapter Seven (see p. 189), and simply add two additional servings of fish, dairy products, legumes, or lean meat during the second and third trimesters, you should be in good shape.

You should eat about 2,200 calories daily in the first trimester, 2,500 in the second and third trimesters, and 2,700 when you're lactating and nursing. Throughout, you should get about 70 grams of protein daily.

## Keep Your Baby Free of Harmful Substances

You should also avoid ingesting anything that might harm your baby, particularly in the first days following conception.

1. *No alcohol.* Fetal alcohol syndrome was identified about twenty years ago, but sadly, many babies today are born with the classic symptoms of this condition. They often have heart abnormalities and mental retardation, and suffer their entire lives because of their mothers' ignorance as to the dangers of alcohol to an embryo when it's conceived.

2. *No caffeine.* Caffeine is a highly addictive stimulant and can also injure the fetus in utero. There are many coffee substitutes made of grain on the market that don't taste like java but have the same warm, delicious effect. You can also drink herbal tea. Overconsumption of caffeine might result in preterm delivery of your baby, or in severe cases, defects in development of the fingers and toes.

3. *No sugar substitutes.* If you have cravings for sugar once in a while, go ahead and indulge them. You don't want to go overboard with sugar (because it provides only empty calories), but it's far less detrimental to your health than saccharin or aspartame, which have proved to cause birth defects in animal studies when consumed in large doses.

4. *No metals, pesticides, or other pollutants.* Mercury poisoning from eating contaminated fish can be dangerous to your baby, as can the fungicide methyl mercury. Your best bet is to limit your fish selections to sole and flounder, which tend to be free of contamination.

## Possible Gastrointestinal Upsets During Pregnancy

Because of your shifting hormones and the realignment of all your internal organs to accommodate the baby within, it's not surprsing that you may suffer at one time or another from a few stomach problems. None of them will endanger you or your baby.

1. *Nausea*. Hormonal changes and the tensions of pregnancy often cause nausea and vomiting, particularly during the first trimester. Sometimes certain food smells can trigger this type of upset, so it may be easier on you if you keep your serious cooking to a minimum for the first couple of months. Nausea is quickly relieved by complex carbohydrates, so keep some low-fat crackers by your bedside and in your purse. You may also want to consume fewer, smaller meals.

2. *Heartburn*. This condition is caused by a regurgitation of stomach acids and a feeling of fullness around the middle of your chest. It is caused partly by the baby displacing the stomach upward, also by the hormonal changes of pregnancy that relax the muscle opening at the top of the stomach and cause it to empty more slowly and to allow stomach acids to enter the gullet.

The burping, sour sensation you get when you have heartburn can be reduced or eliminated by having smaller, more frequent meals, by eating more slowly and chewing more thoroughly.

3. *Constipation*. This condition is caused by the slowing effect of the hormone progresterone on the digestive tract. Another reason for getting constipated is that as your baby grows, the intestines are increasingly displaced and compressed by the uterus, making it harder for digested material to pass through the system.

Never use laxatives; rather, add more fiber to your diet. You can consume whole grains and bran, fruits and vegetables and occasionally, prunes, figs, and all-bran cereals.

4. *Hemorrhoids*. These protruding veins around the opening of the anus are an unfortunate side-effect of constipation. As it becomes

more difficult to pass stool, and you strain to have a bowel movement, you create additional pressure in these veins. They may occasionally rupture and bleed, which is unsettling, but not dangerous.

You should certainly add fiber to your diet to alleviate your constipation; at the same time, you may want to use aloe or witch-hazel preparations, such as Tucks wipes, on your anal area.

## SUPPLEMENTS FOR THE PREGNANT WOMAN

You should, of course, be conservative and cautious about whatever you put into your body at this time. With some vitamins and minerals, it's a good idea to cut back; with others, you need additional supplementation for the healthy development of your fetus.

Your physician or midwife can start you on a prenatal vitamin when you first conceive, and you should take these throughout your pregnancy and lactation. The vitamin pill should contain a good approximation of the ingredients that follow—if it doesn't, ask your healthcare provider if you should take additional amounts.

| | |
|---|---|
| *Vitamin* A: | no more than 5,000 IU daily |
| *Vitamin* B3: | at least 17 mg. daily, but not more than 50 mg. |
| *Vitamin* B6: | at least 2.2 mg. daily |
| *Folic acid*: | 800 mg. daily (more than twice the prepregnant requirement) |
| *Vitamin* C: | 500 to 1,000 mg. daily |
| *Vitamin* D: | 10 mcg. daily |
| *Vitamin* E: | no more than 60 IU daily |
| *Vitamin* K: | 65 mcg. daily |
| *Calcium*: | 1,200 mg. |
| *Magnesium*: | 600 mg. |
| *Iron*: | 30 mg. |

— SIDEBAR I —

## WOMEN'S DAILY RECOMMENDED DOSAGES OF VITAMINS

| Vitamin | Approximate Daily Dosage | |
| --- | --- | --- |
| | *Premenopausal* | *Postmenopausal* |
| $B_1$ | 5 mg. | 2.5 mg. |
| $B_2$ | 5 mg. | 2.5 mg. |
| $B_3$ (niacin) | 100 to 1,000 mg.* | 100 to 1,000 mg.* |
| $B_6$ | 4 mg. | 3 mg. |
| $B_{12}$ | 20 mcg. | 40 mcg. |
| Beta-carotene | 25,000 IU | 25,000 IU |
| Biotin | 210 mcg. | 300 mcg. |
| Choline | 250 mg. | 250 mg. |
| Folic Acid | 300 mcg. | 400 mcg. |
| Inositol | 500 mg. | 500 mg. |
| PABA | 100 mg. | 100 mg. |
| Pantothenic Acid | 30 mg. | 30 mg. |
| C | varies; start with 1 gram | |
| D | 400 IU | 400 IU |
| E | 140 to 600 IU | 180 to 700 IU |

* With your doctor's advice and supervision.

SIDEBAR II

## WOMEN'S DAILY RECOMMENDED DOSAGES OF MINERALS

| Mineral | Approximate Daily Dosage | |
| --- | --- | --- |
| | *Premenopausal* | *Postmenopausal* |
| Calcium | 1,000 mg. | 1,500 mg. |
| Copper | 2 mg. | 3 mg. |
| Chromium | 200 mcg. | 200 mcg. |
| Magnesium | 320 mg. | 300 mg. |
| Manganese | 2 mg. | 5 mg. |
| Molybdenum | 50 mcg. | 50 mcg. |

| | | |
|---|---|---|
| Selenium | 200 mcg. | 200 mcg. |
| Zinc | 15 mg. | 15 mg. |
| Iodine | 150 mcg. | 150 mcg. |
| Potassium | 860 mg. | 860 mg. |

— SIDEBAR III —

## No-Pain Grains

| Grain (1 cup) | Water (cups) | Simmer for | Let Stand | Yield (cups) |
|---|---|---|---|---|
| Amaranth | 3 | 25 min. | 0 min. | 2 |
| Barley (pearled) | 3 | 50 min. | 10 min. | $3^1/_2$ |
| Brown rice | $2^1/_2$ | 45 min. | 10 min. | $3^1/_2$ |
| Buckwheat groats | 2 | 12 min. | 5 min. | 2 |
| Bulgur | 2 | 15 min. | 5 min. | 3 |
| Couscous | 2 | 0 min.* | 10 min. | 3 |
| Millet | 2 | 25 min. | 5 min. | $3^1/_2$ |
| Quinoa | 2 | 15 min. | 5 min. | 3 |
| Triticale** | $2^1/_4$ | $1^3/_4$ hr. | 10 min. | 2 |
| Wheat berries** | $3^1/_2$ | 1 hr. | 15 min. | 2 |
| Wild rice | $2^1/_4$ | 45 min. | 10 min. | $2^1/_2$ |

*Instructions:*

1. Boil the water and add the grain
2. Bring the water back to a boil, cover, and reduce heat to a simmer.
3. After simmering, remove the pot from the burner and let stand, covered.

  \* Put the couscous into a bowl, add the boiling water, cover and let stand.
  \*\* Soak overnight before cooking.

Chart adapted from *Recipes from an Ecological Kitchen,* by Lorna J. Sass (William Morrow and Co., 1992).

— SIDEBAR IV —

## IDEAL WEIGHT FOR WOMEN

| Height | | Frame | | |
| Ft | In | Small | Medium | Large |
|---|---|---|---|---|
| 4 | 10 | 102–111 | 109–121 | 118–131 |
| 4 | 11 | 103–113 | 111–123 | 120–134 |
| 5 | 0 | 104–115 | 113–126 | 122–137 |
| 5 | 1 | 106–118 | 115–129 | 125–140 |
| 5 | 2 | 108–121 | 118–132 | 128–143 |
| 5 | 3 | 111–124 | 121–135 | 131–147 |
| 5 | 4 | 114–127 | 124–138 | 134–151 |
| 5 | 5 | 117–130 | 127–141 | 137–155 |
| 5 | 6 | 120–133 | 130–144 | 140–159 |
| 5 | 7 | 123–136 | 133–147 | 143–163 |
| 5 | 8 | 126–139 | 136–150 | 146–167 |
| 5 | 9 | 129–142 | 138–153 | 149–170 |
| 5 | 10 | 132–145 | 142–156 | 152–173 |
| 5 | 11 | 135–148 | 145–159 | 155–176 |
| 6 | 0 | 138–151 | 148–162 | 158–179 |

Based on a weight-height mortality study conducted by the Society of Actuaries and the Association of Life Insurance Medical Directors of America. Metropolitan Life Insurance Company, revised 1983.

Height includes 1-in. heel. Weight includes 5 pounds for indoor clothing.

— SIDEBAR V —

## FOODS HIGH IN CALCIUM

| Food | Milligrams of Calcium |
|---|---|
| 1 cup of nonfat yogurt | 300 |
| 3 oz. sardines | 320 |
| 1 cup skim milk | 300 |
| 3 oz. salmon | 180 |
| 3 oz. tofu | 175 |
| 1/2 cup collard greens | 150 |
| 1/2 cup cooked spinach | 120 |
| 1/2 cup boiled broccoli | 90 |
| 1/2 cup white beans | 80 |

— SIDEBAR VI —

## THE TOP TEN FOODS HIGH IN VITAMIN C
(In Descending Order)

1. Sweet red, raw bell pepper

2. Papayas

3. Hot red or green, raw chili peppers

4. California navel oranges

5. Cantaloupe

6. Kiwi

7. Florida oranges

8. Broccoli

9. Black currants

10. Sprouts

# EXERCISE
## AWAY THE YEARS

CHAPTER 3

$A$ constant 115 pounds for a five-foot, five-inches frame isn't bad at any age—especially age 67. At this point in her life, physical fitness expert Marjorie Craig said, "I hate the term 'senior citizen.' If human beings feel good, look good, and can carry on their lives, why stick a name on them just because they're ten, twenty or thirty years older than they once were?"

Teaching women from teens up through the 70s how to stay fit, Ms. Craig was a living example of how a commitment to fitness could help keep women looking ten years younger.

And sexier, too! More orgasms for women—27 percent more—according to a study of 8,145 women by Dr. L. DeVillers, if they exercise at least three times a week for three months or more. Forty percent of these same women reported an increase in their ability to be sexually aroused since starting an exercise program. Almost nine out of ten reported an increase in "sexual confidence" and one-third reported increased sexual activity with their partners.

In another study, Dr. Philip Whitten of Harvard University and his colleague, Elizabeth Whiteside, studied male and female swimmers in their 40s and 60s, a total of 160 swimmers in all. On the average, these swimmers swam for about an hour a day, four or five days a week.

Many deviated from this average, however, allowing the researchers to compare intensity of activity with effect on sexuality. Some swam less, others up to three or four hours a day, six days a week. Overall, those in their 40s reported sex lives similar to average people in their 20s and 30s. Swimmers in their 60s reported sex lives similar to those in their 40s.

According to the report: "97 percent of those in their 40s and 92 percent of those in their 60s said they were sexually active—very high compared to what research has suggested about the sex lives of the general population over 40.

"The frequency of intercourse among these swimmers 40 and over was similar to that reported by many people in their 20s and 30s—about seven times a month. And the frequency did not drop off; the swimmers in their 60s were nearly as active as those in their 40s.

"And perhaps even more interesting, spouses and lovers of the swimmers rated them as *even more attractive* than the swimmers rated themselves."

## THREE HOURS A WEEK FOR BETTER SEX

But too much of anything can be bad. For the wonderful results just described, all the training that is needed is just 45 minutes a day, about three days a week. For those who went to extremes—18 or more hours a week—sexual desire began to diminish. In the previous study, Dr. DeVillers found the same thing. So, for a healthy, long-lasting and enjoyable sex life, the basic three hours a week of training is perfectly adequate. More probably won't hurt, until you go to extremes of six times that amount. Certainly, three to ten hours a week should work out just fine, for you *and* your lover.

However, there are caveats. If one member of a couple becomes fit while the other continues a sedentary lifestyle, the latter is susceptible to feeling very insecure about this change of status. As a woman becomes more svelte and active, her sedentary boyfriend may worry. This may be more of a problem with couples that are not married, where people have less of a commitment to one another.

This fear of losing a relationship can become a real obstacle in continuing an otherwise successful training program.

## Trade Love for Exercise Time

To overcome such an obstacle, reassure your lover/spouse about your undying love (if such is true) and negotiate a trade-off where time taken away from the relationship for training will be compensated for in some other form. For example, more loving? Especially if you were to work out together? You get the idea. Be creative in allowing the fitness lifestyle to add to rather than detract from your relationship.

But we're getting ahead of ourselves. What about the basics of fitness? Now that I've used sex to get your attention, let's look at how training for fitness can contribute to adding ten youthful years to your life.

According to the American Heart Association, lack of exercise is one of 11 factors that predispose us to heart disease. And as for our concern about "creeping" overweight, I'm convinced that inactivity is as important a factor as overeating. Unequivocally, exercise slows the aging process. So, for a healthier heart, a slimmer body, and a longer life, try getting off your duff.

I know, you have a good number of convincing reasons not to. You don't have time. You're overstressed with time demands as it is. Why add to the stress by putting more time demands on your life? For there's no getting around the fact that exercise takes time; we even measure it in units of time—a 45-minute workout, 20-minute walk, and so on.

Besides that, exercise is painful and sweaty—how can that be any fun! "Sure," you'd like me to reassure you, "sit back and relax! Life is too short!"

"Made shorter," you won't want me to add, "by the greater inevitability of obesity, coronary disease, high blood pressure and its companion in old age, stroke, and a generally sickly disposition."

Have I talked you into some movement yet? Well, consider this: Heart attacks are the leading cause of death in women. Post-menopausal women are particularly susceptible to heart attack.

# HOW EXERCISE PROLONGS YOUR LIFE

Exercise:

1. Decreases your risk of heart attack.

2. Aids your heart in doing its job more effectively.

3. Helps your body use oxygen more effectively.

4. Improves circulation throughout your body.

5. Lowers blood pressure and cholesterol.

6. Decreases the incidents of hot flashes for menopausal women.

7. Helps you lose weight more effectively by burning fat and raising your metabolism.

8. Makes your muscles both stronger and more elastic.

9. Enhances your immune system (except for a few hours after grueling marathons).

10. Decreases stress and the destructive effects of depression.

## Fourteen Minutes a Day Will Make a Difference

In a 1973 study entitled, "Vigorous Exercise in Leisure Time and the Incidence of Coronary Heart Disease," over 16,000 subjects between the ages of 40 and 64 were studied by the British scientist, J. N. Morris and his colleagues. They compared those who included at least 14 uninterrupted minutes a day of running, swimming or bicycling in their ongoing lifestyle with those who were inactive. Those who reported regular, vigorous exercise in their lives suffered only one-third the number of heart attacks as did their less active counterparts. So, you see, it doesn't take much activity to result in a very important health difference.

In a more thorough investigation of over 500 of these same individuals, electrocardiogram data indicated that the inactive ones showed twice as many heart abnormalities as did the exercising group.

## Active Work Means Fewer Fatal Heart Attacks

Here in America, a long-term study of over 20 years on more than 6,000 San Francisco Bay longshoremen (a study not to be taken light-heartedly) revealed, when all the data were scientifically sorted out to allow for individual differences, that high-energy output on the job substantially *reduced* the risk of fatal heart attack. Less active workers were three times more likely to die of a heart attack than their more active counterparts.

The data also revealed that those who were less active, smoked heavily and had high blood pressure were *twenty* times as likely to suffer a fatal heart attack than their counterparts who had none of these three characteristics.

## How to Be Completely Immune to Heart Disease

At least one scientist believes that it is possible to become entirely immune to heart disease, by increasing the level of activity to a certain criterion. And just what is that specific criterion? According to Dr. Tom Bassler, it is the ability to complete a marathon. Beginning in 1967, Dr. Bassler did an ongoing, worldwide analysis of the deaths of marathon runners. After histological analysis of over 200 such deaths, not one proved to be from heart disease. Responding to challenges from the medical community, Dr. Bassler does submit that such immunity lasts only while the runner is in training.

## Scientific Proof that Exercise Lengthens the Lifespan

What about proof of the effect of exercise on prolonging life? Such research is more attainable from animals than humans, for reasons that begin to become obvious once you think about it. It is much easier to do lifespan research on animals because the researcher is more likely to outlive his subjects. In addition, it would be unethical to manipulate factors in human lives that might end up shortening their lives. So we're more likely to rely on rodents rather than humans for such research. I'll mention only two such studies.

In one (that used male mice only) when mice were allowed to engage in wheel exercise, it was found that they were able to extend their lifespan by 10 percent. Perhaps the exercise didn't start early enough—the mice were almost two years old at the beginning of the study, practically senior citizens in mouse-terms.

A more long-term study, where rats began 10-minute exercise sessions on a motor-driven drum at one month of age (about three years old in human terms), was conducted at Ohio State University. In this lifelong study, the lifespan of the exercising rats proved to be 31 percent longer than their relatively less active counterparts. This time, both males and females were equally affected.

So this research implies that if we start early, exercise can lengthen our lifespans considerably. But even if we begin as senior citizens, we can still aspire to an added few years of productive life.

## Combine Exercise with Decreased Food Intake

Losing weight through a combination of reducing food consumption and increasing exercise is superior to losing weight through food reduction alone. With exercise, more body fat is lost with virtually no loss of muscle tissue.

# DR. RYBACK'S SPEAR METHOD FOR GETTING STARTED

If you happen to be a sedentary type, it is extremely important that you have a medical checkup as well as a fitness evaluation prior to starting your exercise regimen. Your doctor will most likely take a medical history, including questions about illness in your family, and perform a physical exam, including a blood analysis and an electrocardiogram. If you're over 40, an exercise treadmill study or stress test will pick up any apparent heart problems.

## The SPEAR Approach to Getting Started

For getting started (or restarted), allow me to share an acronym I've used for myself: SPEAR.

**S** - **S**et a goal: Losing five pounds, fitting into your tight clothes, winning a trophy, running a marathon.

**P** - **P**ick an exercise you like, one that is compatible with your schedule, that fits into your life logistically (near a park, pool, or airport).

**E** - **E**njoy. Not only should you enjoy the activity itself, but allow music, the right companion(s), and sense of competition to fulfill their roles. When running, I enjoy anticipating the Saturday morning road races. When swimming, I enjoy the company of other swimmers at the pool. To each his own—find your own.

**A** - **A**lways do your exercise. Make it a high priority in your daily schedule. Don't allow exceptions to become the rule. I discipline myself by not having my dinner until I've done my run or swim. I usually end up running when I get hungry enough.

**R** - **R**outine is extremely helpful. If I'm running, I make sure my running gear is handy and my Walkman batteries are recharged, so when the time comes, I won't have to mess with those things and become distracted. With swimming, I make sure I have my goggles and dry swimsuit handy when the time comes. If you can do your activity the same time each day, all the better. The more routine the logistics, the easier you'll make it for yourself.

## CUSTOMIZE YOUR WORKOUT

When it comes to workouts, never has the phrase "different strokes for different folks" been more apt. Depending on your age, weight, energy level, schedule and budget, you may choose one activity over another. To assist you in this decision-making process, a chart follows which should help you pick the best activity for you.

Based on your age, energy level and body type, this chart suggests activities you might choose as starting points. As you progress, be flexible in trying new activities, as your schedule and budget allow and as your interests guide you.

Here are some guidelines, according to your body type:

## Ectomorphs

If you've got a tendency to remain thin, you're probably high in energy with above-average endurance. Chances are you eat more than most women, yet remain quite slim.

Since you tend to be light in muscle as well as fat, I recommend weight training for all age levels and all energy levels. Since your light weight makes you vulnerable to injury in team sports, I recommend that only for those women with higher energy levels.

Since I recommend weight training for ectomorphs at all ages and energy levels, I want to share some general guidelines to help you get started. I'll assume you will want to build a sexy figure rather quickly so you can see some visible results from all your efforts.

1. Focus on your exercise program, not on socializing. It's tempting to "hang out" and banter with other men and women about what you're doing to build your figure. Your time is limited. Do what you've come to do and get the job done. It takes a lot of repetitions (reps) to get those muscles bulging.

2. Be sure to drink your 8 glasses of water daily. You'll especially need this as your muscles begin to fill out your figure.

3. Warm up with each exercise by going through the motions with a very light weight. Then immediately go to the heaviest weight of which you're capable, and fatigue your muscles by doing as many reps as you can. For your second set, decrease the weights by 5 to 15 pounds or whatever weight it takes for you to complete 8 to 10 reps before your muscles are fatigued. Keep experimenting along these lines until you're selecting the right weights for this "count-down" procedure. Then just watch your muscles tone up.

## Mesomorphs

If you have a good figure without much fat on a medium build, running, aerobics, and cycling are good activities for most of you. The loss in weight you might achieve through running and cycling too, may be right for you. Your well-centered body type makes aerobics a good choice for those of you who are more energetic.

### Endomorphs

With a tendency to put on weight, swimming is a great start for you, first, because your body type will give you buoyancy in the water, and second, because you need the intensity of swimming exercise to transform some of that fat into a more shapely figure.

I don't recommend running as a starting point for you because the extra weight may damage your knees or other joints.

The following chart will help you find the most appropriate fitness activities for your age, body build, and energy level.

| AGE | Ectomorph | | | Mesomorph | | | Endomorph | | |
|-----|-----|-----|-----|-----|-----|-----|-----|-----|-----|
| Over 20 | WT | WC | IW | RT | RT | IC | SW | ST | IC |
| Over 40 | WT | WC | IW | TC | TC | IC | SW | SC | IS |
| Over 60 | SW | SW | SW | SW | SW | SW | SW | SW | IW |
| Energy level | high | med | low | high | med | low | high | med | low |

KEY:

C = Cycling
I = Individual activities
R = Running
S = Swimming
T = Team sports
W = Weight lifting

---

## BE YOUR OWN PERSONAL TRAINER: SIX TIPS FOR STICKING TO A WORKOUT PROGRAM

---

1. *Begin slowly and build gradually.* If you start with walking or jogging, use your THR to guide you. Whatever you do, it's terribly important that you begin very slowly and increase your intensity very, very gradually. The worst thing you can do is try too hard initially and burn yourself out before allowing your form of exercise to become a habit.

2. *Walk with friends or music.* If you're walking, explore different routes if you can. Do all you can to make the walk enjoyable. A Walkman with your favorite music or an interesting and equally devoted companion will do wonders to make this activity enjoyable. And it must be enjoyable if it's going to last.

3. *Run for the glory.* Music or a companion will also help jogging. As you slowly build your distance, you can begin exploring the possibility of joining the many Saturday morning friendly walks and runs that offer small trophies and T-shirts if you compete successfully in your age group.

4. *How to deal with bad weather.* If you're a walker and you don't live in a safe area or you don't like bad weather (hot or cold), you can drive to your city airport (or mall) and walk indoors.

5. *The secret to successful exercising.* Whatever your choice, try to exercise the same time every day. Otherwise, everything else will take priority and your exercise will fall between the cracks. Some women enjoy getting up earlier than usual and completing their exercise to start their day. Others will use their lunch hour and reward themselves with a light lunch (yogurt and fruit, for example) and have an alert, productive afternoon while their well-fed colleagues struggle to stay awake on a full belly. Still others prefer to wait until the end of the day and use their exercise time to unwind from the stresses of the day. Whatever time you choose, make it consistent, so that there's no decision to make at the time. In my opinion, that's the secret to successful aerobic exercising.

6. *Have the best accessories.* As for equipment, this is one aspect of your life in which you need to be good to yourself. Get the best walking or running shoes you can afford. And get good advice from a knowledgeable salesperson at the time of purchase. For swimming, all you need is a good pair of swim goggles and probably a rubber swim cap. Oh, and don't forget the swimsuit, unless you have a private pool.

# SEVEN BACK-STRENGTHENING EXERCISES

If you want to strengthen your back, make a commitment to 15 minutes a day during which you can do each of the following exercises five times. Do this 3 to 5 days a week. If you have a bad back, check with your doctor first.

1. Lie on your stomach with elbows bent by your sides and hands flat on the floor. Keeping your hips on the floor, slowly lift your upper body until you feel a slight stretch in your lower back. Hold for 15 seconds.

2. In the same position, place a small pillow under your stomach. With your arms held against your sides, raise your head and shoulders just off the floor. Count to 5, then gradually lower yourself.

3. In the same position, keeping arms extended straight above your head, raise your right arm and left leg and hold for a count of 5. Then repeat with your left arm and right leg.

4. Turn over on your back, placing the pillow under the small of your back, and bend one knee while keeping the other flat on the floor. Grab the bent leg just behind the knee and pull gently toward your chest until you feel the gentle pull in your lower back. Repeat for the other leg.

5. Repeat this with both legs, rolling your shoulders forward, tucking your chin to your chest and lifting your shoulders a few inches off the floor.

6. In the same position, bend both knees with your feet flat on the floor, and your arms, palms down, along your sides. Lift your head and shoulders gently off the floor and hold for a count of five. Return and rest for at least 10 seconds before repeating.

## EXERCISE FOR BETTER SEX

We get better with practice, and that goes for sex as it does for anything else. Men, usually (but not always), are the more active in sexual positioning and movement while women are typically more receptive, but even that takes physical fitness. So here are some exercises that will put you in excellent form for better sex.

Working from the top down, muscles important to sexual fitness are the arms (the better to hold you, my dear), abdominals (for better thrust), hips and groin (where the action is).

### 1. Arms

The trick is not only to achieve strength in the arms, which you get from lifting weights and other upper body exercise, but also flexibility. Rolling around in the hay requires flexibility.

For best results, straighten your arms in front of you, grab your left wrist with your right hand and extend your arms up above your head and slightly backward until you feel the gentle pull under your armpits. Hold for a count of 5, then relax your arms, and repeat once or twice.

### 2. Abdominals

Perhaps the most important muscles for a woman's lovemaking, the abdominals, can be strengthened by well-known crunches. Lying on your back with knees bent, and arms folded across your chest or clasped behind your neck for support, slowly bring your head and shoulders up until your shoulders are 4 inches off the floor. Hold for a count of 3, then relax and repeat, as often as you feel comfortable. Slowly increase the number as you get familiar with this exercise.

### 3. Hips and Groin

Flexibility is the key here rather than strength. Two exercises can help you attain this.

First, seated on the floor with your feet together and bent knees apart, reach for your ankles with your elbows between your knees.

Now grasp your ankles and allow your soles to come together against one another. Bend forward slightly as you allow the pressure of your elbows against your knees to force your knees down toward the floor ever so gently. When you feel the pull in your groin, stop and hold for a few seconds. Relax your hold and repeat two or three times, making sure to be very gentle.

For the second, sit with your legs crossed and lean forward slightly with your arms stretched out in front of you. When you feel the pull in your groin, lean into it very gently once or twice more. Relax and repeat 2 or 3 times.

### 4. Kegel Exercises

First discovered in the '40s by Dr. Arnold Kegel in order to help women gain better bladder control, these exercises can also help you attain more intense orgasms more often.

The muscles in focus here are those that control the flow of urine. There are three basic exercises, and all are fairly simple to describe, if not to carry out. In the first, imagine your intention to stop the flow of urine once it has begun. You can feel the muscle deep within your groin tense up. Do this and hold for a count of three. Over time, you can increase the count to five and then ten as you're comfortably progressing.

For the second exercise, clench and relax these same muscles as quickly as you can.

For the third exercise, imagine forcing out the last drops of urine after voiding your bladder. This time you'll feel your abdominal walls tighten up as well.

Complete 10 slow reps of each of these exercises approximately 5 times a day. After a while, you'll feel more sensitive and in control of your orgasms. Some women can also attain longer-lasting orgasms once they become proficient in these exercises.

## PUSHING 90, PUMPING IRON

Weight lifting has been shown to prolong life by slowing down or eliminating the effects of such diseases as arthritis, lung disease, and other conditions, even for 90-year-olds. One recent study of 50 frail, elderly nursing home residents in their 80s and 90s surveyed the effects of hip and knee resistance exercises. The result of 10 weeks of these exercise regimens three times a week was greater strength and muscle size, as well as improved mobility and more spontaneous activity.

Take, Sol, for instance. At 91 years of age, he was limited to shuffling along slowly to keep up with his younger wife Celia, a sprightly 82 years of age. A lack of exercise kept Sol looking and feeling disabled. Once he began a comfortable regimen of easy leg exercises, he felt more comfortable climbing stairs without assistance and keeping up with his youthful wife. Enjoying their golden years together, Sol and Celia could now be seen together during their daily sojourns, arm in arm, enjoying the afternoon sun. Pushing 92, Sol is now able to enjoy his youthful wife even more fully.

## GETTING BACK INTO SHAPE AFTER PREGNANCY

It can be disheartening to look in the mirror after delivering your baby and see a body that still looks pregnant. Nature has designed the female to hold onto a considerable amount of weight after birth as preparation for nursing. In centuries past, it was vital to a woman's survival that she retain at least ten extra pounds over her prepregnancy weight so that she would have the strength and stamina to care for a new life.

It is equally important for modern women to have additional fat cells that will sustain them through breastfeeding. But it still makes you feel rotten when you expected to nurse in your size 10 jeans and, instead, have to wear your maternity pants. And if you're having a baby later in life, your body isn't as elastic as it used to be. It is common for mothers over 35 to find that even when they do get back to their prepregnancy weight, they have a larger waist and bigger hips.

One of my patients, Eva, was suffering badly from postpartum depression. She saw me several weeks after giving birth and confided that her husband seemed to have transferred all his love to their new baby girl. Although she wanted her husband to bond with the baby, she hadn't expected to feel so left out. "Is this normal?" she asked me tearfully. "Maybe it's because I'm so fat. I expected to bounce right back to my old figure, but look at me. I've never been this heavy in my entire life."

Eva's distress is all too common, and our society, which worships the skinny women we see daily on TV, in film, and in magazine ads, reinforces her self-deprecating feelings. Of course, it isn't just body image that can cause postpartum depression. There are many factors, chief among which is the terrifying thought that your life now revolves around this small, dependent, hungry being. You also have to reestablish your relationship with your partner and to bring this new life into your already existing family. It can sometimes feel as though you're the only one in the world that has ever gone through this experience.

But it's easier to focus on the blatant weight problem, and that's the one that seems to give most new mothers the "baby blues." Getting back in shape after pregnancy is particularly challenging today because we expect new mothers to be superwomen. They have to race back from the hospital with barely a day to recuperate from the birth experience to get their household into gear. Many have to return to the workplace within six weeks or forfeit their jobs. It's almost impossible *not* to fall into the trap of believing that you can do it all: give birth, clinch a new deal, get a promotion, and appear at the dinnertable looking ravishing—and thin. The truth of the matter is that the average woman will retain about two pounds per baby, even after she's back in shape.

If you go easy on yourself and don't expect miracles, you should be able to see some changes within a few weeks. Your postpartum depression should lessen as time passes and your hormones get back in balance. If they don't, and if you find that you are unable to find any delight in your life—including holding your new baby— some short-term counseling may be in order.

For most women, however, this should be a smooth passage. Here are some tips for getting back in physical and mental shape:

## 1. Relax and Give Yourself Two Weeks as a Transition

You've been growing steadily along with your baby for the past nine months. In China, the belief goes that a woman deserves another nine months to return to herself. So you can certainly spare two weeks to just lie back and get to know your child and let others do for you. If you make no demands on your body other than feeding and caring for your child, it will respond in kind.

Breastfeeding is a definite plus for mother and child. Breast milk is, bar none, the best nutrition a newborn can have. It contains every nutrient, vitamin, and mineral, and provides adequate hydration, as well. It will protect your baby from potential allergies and illnesses, and will help you get back into shape because nursing actually increases your metabolism.

Many nursing mothers find that they can eat heartily and lose weight because of the increased energy needs of their bodies. Even if you don't lose, you will find that as you get back to being your prepregnant self and can start exercising again, your body will start to regain a semblance of its former shape.

### 2. Exercises for the First Six Weeks

As long as your obstetrician or midwife agrees, there's no reason why you shouldn't start some gentle stretching right away. Remember that your *lochia* (the vaginal discharge tinged with blood) that flows for about six weeks, will be pretty heavy at this time. Excess physical activity will cause you to flow more heavily, which is why you shouldn't jump right back into your regular exercise routine. Take it slowly, and at the end of this transition period, you'll be ready for more.

Try these exercises to help smooth the transition period:

❒ Lie on your back and bring one knee up, cradling it in your arms. Bring your head up to touch your knee. Hold for a few seconds, let it down, then repeat on the other side. Do five repetitions on each side.

❒ Lie on your back and bend your knees, bringing them close to your body so that your heels nearly touch your buttocks. Cross your arms over your chest and bring your head and shoulders up toward your knees. Hold for a few seconds, then lower your head slowly. Repeat five times.

❒ Lie on your back and bend your knees, bringing them close to your body so that your heels nearly touch your buttocks. Place your arms at your side, palms down and press down to bring your buttocks off the floor. Support your weight equally on your shoulders, hands and feet. Repeat twice.

❐ Stand up and as you bend at the waist, begin to round your body over, letting your arms drop straight down. Go only as far as you can comfortably—don't bounce or try to touch your toes. Each day, set yourself a goal of moving down a little further, first to the knees, then the ankles, then the tops of your feet.

At the end of six weeks postpartum, you should be ready to start the yoga exercises in Chapter Four (see p. 119). Move slowly at first and progress at your own pace. *Remember, this is not a race!* Whenever you get back in shape, that's the time that's right for you.

In the next few months, you can go back to your regular fitness routine. You can and should exercise daily. Ask your partner, friend, or relative to watch the baby while you go out and get yourself back into shape.

### 3. Drink Plenty of Fluids

You cannot overdo on your consumption of water, low-fat milk, juices, and herbal teas. If you're nursing, double the amount you would ordinarily drink. You might like to keep a glass of milk beside you as you nurse so you can get enough liquid and nutrition at the same time.

### 4. Eat Right and Don't Worry About Weight Loss

Make sure you have a well-rounded diet and enough calcium intake, particularly if you're nursing. Eat lots of dairy (low-fat milk and yogurt) and fish *with* bones (sardines, mackerel, and salmon) as well as sole and flounder, two fishes that are relatively pollutant-free. For adequate potassium, don't forget to have a daily banana. Eat whole grain breads and pastas, bran cereal, brown rice, and plenty of legumes (beans, peas, and lentils). If you don't think you have time to cook, keep a good assortment of salad fixing around, which you can always sprinkle with sunflower seeds, raisins, and wheat germ.

### 5. Avoid Sugar and Excess Salt

Sugar simply contains empty calories and gives you no nutritive value. Although a candy bar or cupcake may give you a burst of energy, the down side is that an hour later, your blood sugar drops dramatically and you may feel fatigued once again. A piece of whole wheat toast with apple butter will give you the same lift in the middle of the day and its effects will last much longer, and will keep your blood sugar at an even keel.

Although you need some salt in your diet, particularly if you're nursing, too much will cause you to retain fluids and feel bloated. So salt can add to a weight problem.

## 6. Reach for Your Goals

As the months go by and you become acclimated to parenthood, try to keep a regular eating and exercise routine. All the good resolutions you make right after you give birth are easy to forget once life gets back to normal. But if you review this chapter, you'll be reminded of your commitment to living ten years longer and looking ten years younger, and what better time to prepare for that than just after you've brought a new life into the world?

In order to stick to your personal longevity program, you will need to recruit your partner, family, and friends so that you never have a day where you don't do some yoga, exercise, or meditation. Consider taking your infant along when you exercise. You can take a brisk walk with your baby in a backpack, or jog with her as she rides in her three-wheeled running stroller. (These are available in most baby furniture stores and in many sports equipment and baby catalogues.) If you sign up for a health club or gym, make sure they have child-care services.

Nothing is impossible! If you're a healthy person, you're a healthy parent. So staying in shape will benefit both you and your child.

Here are my Ten Commandments for staying fit forever:

## STAYING FIT FOREVER

1. Find an activity you enjoy.
2. Find friends to join you in this activity.
3. Begin slowly, build gradually.
4. Exercise to music for an extra burst of energy.

5. Exercise at the same time every day.

6. Exercise daily, or at the very least, do a minimum of 30 to 45 minutes three days a week.

7. Vary your workout to keep it fresh.

8. Eat smaller portions of more healthful foods.

9. Allow your newfound delight in your body to spark your sexual interest.

10. Make your commitment stronger as the years go by.

By continuing to stay active as you get older, you'll be able to add healthy years to your life. Success begets success, and physical activity begets fitness. The more you challenge yourself to take part in a regimen of enjoyable exercise, the more you'll be turning back the clock.

— SIDEBAR I —

## DETERMINING YOUR TARGET HEART RATE

Aerobic exercise, done for at least 30 minutes, stimulates the entire body and reaches maximum effect as you reach your *Target Heart Rate* (THR). This often appears to be a complicated procedure to figure out numerically. So let's take a few minutes now to master this and get it out of the way.

Start with the number 220. Subtract your age. Now from that figure subtract your resting heart rate (usually between 60 and 80). Since you're a beginner, multiply the new number by 60 percent. To that, add your resting heart rate. The number you now have is your THR. Divide that by 6, so that you can take your pulse for 10 seconds to see if you've reached your THR.

It's worthwhile going through a theoretical example to make sure you've got it right. Once you have it, you can use it for a long time. Let's assume you're 40 and that your resting heart rate is 70.

Step 1   220 – 40 (age) = 180

Step 2   180 – 70 (resting heart rate) = 110

Step 3   110 × 60% (for beginners) = 66

Step 4    66 + 70 (resting heart rate) = 136

Step 5   136 ÷ 6 (ten-sec. interval) = 22 or 23

Now when you exercise, you can take your pulse for 10 seconds to see how close you've come to your THR. Your THR is your ideal goal. If you're below it, you can push yourself harder. If you're above, slow down for a while.

— SIDEBAR II —

## THE TV WORKOUT

### THREE REASONS WE EAT WHILE WATCHING TV

There may be psychological reasons why so many people eat while watching television. Here's what I think:

1.  While sitting still for extended hours, the body has a compensating tendency to be active. Since we don't move around much while watching TV, one compatible "activity" is eating.

2.  A second reason may be that watching TV is, more than being passive, a receptive modality. That is, we are "taking in" the entertainment before us. Consequently, "taking in" food is in the same modality, and therefore the temptation to eat is very seductive at the time. (The same reasoning applies to eating snacks during movies. Movie theaters make as much, if not more, on popcorn, candy, and soft drinks as they do on the tickets themselves.)

3.  A third reason has to do with the preponderance of TV commercials that sell food products. These serve to make us very susceptible to accompanying our TV watching with eating behaviors. Even now, I still find it hard to resist these temptations while watching TV.

One solution that has worked very well for me is to arrange my living room in such a way that I have some exercise apparatus next to the sofa in front of the TV so that I can easily move to it and become active instead of filling my mouth with food. For me, it really feels as if the exercise is an effective substitute for the activity of eating. As a matter of fact, it would be ideal to have a few exercise options to provide a variety, so you won't get bored with just one. For example, it would be great to have an exercycle, a rowing machine, and some barbells. That way, you could switch from one to the other as you like. This has the obvious advantage of not only avoiding too much snacking but also getting your body fit at the same time.

# ANTIAGING
## STRESS REDUCERS

## CHAPTER 4

Whether you are a mother of three who runs a business out of her house, a single parent with a full-time job, a vice president in a high-pressure corporation, or a divorced woman looking for new direction, you've got stress. If you are determined to live ten years longer, you must actively control the stress in your life.

As destructive as poor nutrition, lack of exercise, smoking or alcoholism, stress erodes body, mind and spirit until finally, it can do its share of damage. Although it's impossible for busy women to eliminate stress from their lives completely, there are many things you can do to reduce the types of stress you're under and to manage and control them more effectively.

## WHAT IS STRESS?

Imagine walking down a city street, and suddenly hearing a lion roaring close by. You would experience what is known as the *fight or flight response*. Your brain would immediately begin to pour out chemicals that would alert your adrenal glands to secrete the stress hormones *adrenalin*, *noradrenalin*, and *cortisol*. These in turn would start your heart racing and blood pressure soaring. Your respiration would speed up, muscles tense, pupils dilate (all the better to see the predator), and your salivary and intestinal secretions would decrease because it's less important for your body to swallow or digest and more important to muster all its resources to escape this danger. You might also have a knot in your stomach, damp palms, wobbly knees, and dry mouth.

However, if you'd been in a *zoo* and heard that lion roar, you wouldn't have blinked an eye. None of the physiological reactions described above would have taken place because you wouldn't have been stressed at all. You would be assured that the lion was at a safe distance and you weren't in any danger at all. What a difference!

And yet, just *thinking* about that lion loose in the street years later could cause a stress reaction as violent as the actual event.

Stress is a psychophysiological reaction to events in our lives, and whether we feel anxious or perfectly calm depends on our interpretation of those events. If we're laid back and just let problems roll off our back, we don't suffer much from stress. The more sensitive we are to life's problems, the more our nervous system is tuned to react and the harder it is for us to restore homeostasis after the alarm stage of the stress has passed.

Over the course of a single day, you might have an upsetting phone call, a near traffic accident, a slew of bills arriving in the mail, and an argument with your partner. All of these unpleasant occurrences happening one after another would keep your levels of stress hormone high.

Or, you might experience the opposite situation—a stretch of time with no calls, nothing happening and life becoming acutely boring. If this social vacuum exists for years (as it often does with older people in our society), it can be devastating. You can be just as stressed by social deprivation and understimulation as you are by high anxiety.

If you don't know how to cope with stress and to relax in the face of worries and problems, you may be shortening your lifespan without even being aware of how much damage you're doing. If, on the other hand, you learn some easy tools to manage the difficult moments of each day, you'll be well on your way to feeling happier in general and maybe even adding a decade to your life.

## Understanding the General Adaptation Syndrome

Hans Selye, the father of stress research, discovered when he was a medical student in 1926 that all individuals who considered themselves "sick," no matter what their illnesses, exhibited a similar set of symptoms. Whether they were depressed or agitated about their condition, they had a feeling of hopelessness and helplessness that kept them from recovering. They seemed too tired to muster the strength to get well.

Selye also discovered a particular chronological sequence in the stress syndrome, which he called the *general adaptation syndrome*. During the first stage, *alarm*, the body shows general stress arousal as the brain and adrenal glands begin to pump out stress hormones. That uneasy feeling tells us that something is wrong and makes us want to either fight or flee.

In the second stage, *resistance*, one body system is most affected by stress. Usually, the most active system is affected—some of us will typically get a headache when we're stressed; others of us will develop tense muscles in the neck, jaw or back; others will suffer stomach-ache, diarrhea or constipation; still others will break out in a rash.

The third and final stage is what Selye called *exhaustion*. At this point the body has used up all its resources and the system that has been resisting breaks down, leading to a malfunction, such as heart attack, cancer, or even death.

The wonderful thing about the human organism is that we keep adapting. But sometimes we don't adapt well enough. However there are proven ways to learn to stop the stress response at the alarm or resistance stages—and that's what you'll learn to do in this chapter.

## How the Body Responds to Stress

When some external event over which you have no control makes you feel pressured and anxious, your brain puts your body on red alert. As your brain and central nervous system pump out "fight or flight" stress hormones, your cardiovascular system goes into high gear, pumping and clotting blood at a faster than normal rate. Women who live under constant high stress are seven times more likely to suffer from coronary artery disease than their less stressed friends and are two to three times more prone to heart attacks.

Your musculoskeletal and nervous systems are also affected, causing cramping and tension throughout the body. I'm sure you know highly stressed people who live in a state of chronic pain, unable to let go of all the tension they carry around.

Probably the most harmful effect of stress on the body is its depressing effect on the immune system. The set of protective mechanisms that allow us to fight disease can be thrown off radically by the stress hormones secreted by our adrenal glands. The hormone *cortisol* appears to block T-cell receptors and therefore slows down the good work of the white blood cells that usually protect us. We simply don't have as many antibodies circulating in our blood and lymph systems to take care of our  illnesses. Women who are under stress suffer more colds, headaches, stomach-aches, sleep disorders, asthma attacks and are more prone to serious illness such as heart disease and cancers.

## Stress Hormones and Your Heart

More women die from heart disease in America than from any other cause. The more stress you have, the more precarious the health of your heart. When you get furious at your teenage daughter or lose your job and feel like no one will ever hire you again, your heart rate, stroke volume, cardiac output and blood pressure all rise dramatically. Your level of LDL cholesterol goes up, encouraging plaque to collect on your artery walls. This also  causes red blood cells to clump together—a dangerous precursor to a heart attack. In the stress response, blood is also diverted away from the liver and intestines. If the liver doesn't get its appropriate supply of blood, it can't do its job of removing toxins and processing fats and sugars as well. Therefore, such substances remain in the blood and are deposited along the walls of the arteries. This can lead to cardiovascular illness if it continues over years. In this way, stress erodes our bodies over time unless we take charge.

## Stress Isn't All Bad

Sally, one of my long-time patients, told me that she wouldn't want to live without stress—it's what makes her get up in the morning, what gives her that oomph and desire to do more and achieve more. What Sally's talking about is *eustress*, or good stress, as opposed to the destructive *dis-stress* we all have to cope with.

If you're involved in a big corporate merger, moving from one state to another and making plans to get married at the same time, you are carrying an incredible amount of *eustress*. The reason it's beneficial stress is that it is short-term and the outcome is generally assumed to be terrific. Eustress helps us to make positive changes in our lives; however, it still creates some stress hormones in the body. But just as we can modify our reaction to distress by learning relaxation techniques and devising new management skills, we can also make eustress work for us by becoming more aware of how it affects us and by getting a better perspective on what to do about it.

# WOMEN AND STRESS

The more challenges you take on, the greater chance you have of feeling overwhelmed. In our society, women are more likely to have been taught that they have to be perfect and to please everyone else before themselves.

If you are a mother, wife, member of the workforce, child of an elderly parent, volunteer at your local church or community center, mentor to a younger person at work or in your neighborhood, member of several committees, and participant in some hobby or sport, you are wearing too many hats. Too many roles to play, too many obligations, and too little time. All this is a recipe for high stress, particularly characteristic of women.

A variety of studies on changing family roles reveals that, even with dual-career couples, the woman is more likely to be in charge of childcare, housecare and parent-care than her male partner. Whereas his levels of stress hormone are highest at the office and then decline (after his commute home, of course!), her levels stay fairly high throughout the day. She leaves one high-stress job, merely to come home to her next one.

Even in households where men share the work, they tend to pitch in with jobs that can be done at any time, such as child care, lawn mowing or tax preparation. Womens' tasks, from shopping for food to preparing meals to taking kids to the doctor in an emergency, tend to be tied to the clock. Since there's no time for a breather, stress is constantly high. Such prolonged, protracted stress in many diverse areas is what puts women at risk for physical illness and emotional depression.

## How Does Stress Affect Different Personalities?

Personalities are as unique as fingerprints, including the full range of feelings and reactions. But there are certain predominant traits that either predispose us to, or protect us from, stress. Here are three basic personality types—A, B, and E—with their own drawbacks and benefits.

TYPE A. Early research on heart disease and stress has identified certain individuals as Type A, competitive, driving, and aggressive. These traits were formerly associated with high achieving, high-testosterone men. But we now know that women are just as likely to be Type As. If you are driven to succeed, can't bear to wait in line, finish other people's sentences, or feel that no one can do the job right except you, you are probably Type A. Generally, such a person has a strong need to control herself and her environment. She competes hotly with her peers and feels she must do more, faster and better than anyone else. She has an intense need to achieve, but she's not always sure *what*. Finally, she is plagued by polyphasic thinking—taking on many tasks at once instead of concentrating on the appropriate one at any particular time.

A Type A woman can fall into the high-stress trap of anger and hostility, but she has a number of good qualities as well. She thrives on eustress, is self-confident about her abilities, and is a true leader, somebody others look up to and follow.

TYPE B. The easy-going, worry-free woman who can let things ride is known as a *Type* B. Calm, cool, and collected, she always feels confident, and that she'll get where she needs to be in time. If not, she expects others will wait for her. She's not as concerned with image as she is with expressing her needs assertively. Because she isn't a control freak, she is less prone to stress-related disease. She is generally patient with others, a good judge of social circumstances, and what we might call an "evolver" rather than a doer. Things come easily to her, and she may deal with them if and when she pleases. Because she doesn't seem pressured—about time, work, money, relationships—she is quite likely to cause stress in the Type As with whom she deals daily.

On the down side, she may not be a great achiever. Because she isn't driven by the challenge of eustress, she may just sit back and allow life to pass her by. Ironically, she may feel chronically understimulated by her environment; she may end up disappointed and just as stressed as her highly driven sister.

TYPE E. Psychologist Harriet Braiker defines the *Type* E woman as one who has to do "everything for everybody." She feels responsible for the world—and acts as caretaker to her partner, her parents, her children, her clubs and organizations, her boss, and her friends. She has a chronic inability to say "no," even after all her time is already accounted for.

Self-sacrificing to a fault, this person is extremely put-upon. Feeling she has to accomplish all this in order to be liked, she gets on edge and may react in passive-aggressive ways. For example, she may bend over backwards preparing an anniversary celebration for her boss and his wife, but somehow forget to send the invitations and end up having to call everyone at the last moment.

The biggest drawback to being a Type E is having no control over one's life because of allowing others to control it. The woman who allows herself to be manipulated by life often develops a "carcinogenic" personality—she may actually be predisposed to developing cancer because of the belief that she is helpless and dependent on others. Her submission to constant pressure and her craving to be perfect may finally do her in.

## Combatting the "Superwoman" Syndrome

Whether you are a Type A, B or E, or a little of each at different times in your life, you can take steps to alleviate the stress that comes with the territory of being a woman. You don't have to be "Superwoman," no matter how many roles you play. You can take a break once in a while and realize that others are as competent as you and can fend for themselves. It's difficult enough being a working mother in a dual-career marriage, being a divorced single mother, or having no children but managing a business and a home at the same time. You don't have to feel put upon each minute of every day.

In order to have a better perspective on what stresses you, you need to learn the difference between rational and irrational thinking. For instance:

1. *Irrational thought*: If I don't agree to move across the country so my husband can take another job, our marriage will break up and I'll be alone for the rest of my life.

2. *Rational counterthought*: A new job isn't as important to him as our family's general wellness and our good marriage. He's not going to chuck his whole life any more than I would mine. We can discuss the pros and cons of moving together and work out a solution.

Doesn't the problem seem much clearer and less threatening when you look at it in a clear-headed manner? There are a variety of powerful tools you can use to change your perspective on stressful situations.

## Learning to Own Your Anger and Use It Constructively

Women often receive mixed messages about their feelings, especially when they're very young. Although it's considered "feminine" to be emotional, only certain emotions are permitted. Sure, little girls can get weepy or ecstatic, but they're not supposed to get angry. It's not nice to make a fuss and yell. Instead, little girls are encouraged to be passive and compliant, to take whatever comes their way and make the best of it.

But years of suppressing anger can harden hearts, quite literally. The blocked feelings that can't find expression may parallel the amount of plaque inside a woman's arteries.

What can you do to take charge of your anger, to express it appropriately, not fearing it but also not letting it take over? One method is to change your focus of control. If you allow the actions of others to affect you personally, you've put the control in their hands. But if you remove your ego from it and just look at the resolution of any dispute as a task to be overcome, you have taken the focus of control back into your own hands. By using positive instead of negative energy, you can use your angry feelings for the general good of all. You'll also be reducing your muscle tension and cardiovascular pressure and perhaps saving yourself from illness.

If you are in a partnered relationship, when arguments crop up, use your anger constructively. The research on fighting with your mate shows that too much or too little can be bad for your health. If you hold in too much, this means that one or both of you are suppressing feelings. This in turn can contribute to high blood pressure and, over time, lead to cardiovascular problems. If you let go too much, you might end up yelling, screaming and hitting. In a relationship where physical violence becomes a daily possibility, the mental and physical health of the couple are in serious jeopardy. Abusive marriages are too commonplace in today's society, in part because too few have been taught to deal well with anger or to use it for good, assertive communication.

The key to better health and longer life is knowing the deeper emotions within yourself, knowing those of your partner, and talking together. The more constructive the talk, the better you'll feel, especially when it comes to dealing with anger. You can argue some, because that gets both points of view out into the open. But you must learn to argue well.

## How to Have an Argument

1. Slow down and air your feelings one at a time.

2. Listen closely when your partner is talking and ask questions if you don't understand the other person's perspective.

3. Give each other the well-deserved luxury of undivided attention. Unplug the phone, close the door, and if you have children at home, ask them for some private time.

4. Don't place blame. Instead of saying, "You did this to me," say, "I felt this way when this happened—how did you feel?"

5. Accept your own weaknesses and build on your strengths. Take responsibility for your own actions and desires.

6. When arguing becomes too intense or hurtful, take time out. You can establish a code word or make the "T" sign for time out.

7. If you'd like your partner to change a certain behavior, explain why it affects you a certain way. You might say, "When you do X to me, it makes me feel Y. Would you consider Z?"

8. Don't wait too long to have an argument. Get your feelings out before they escalate and become too hot to handle.

9. Treat each other with respect. Remember you wouldn't be having fights unless you really cared about one another.

## Stress in the Workplace

No matter what your career, whether you are white, pink, or blue collar, or if you've reached the glass ceiling and are attempting to crash right through it, you've got stress on the job. Research has shown that women's major work stress is lack of control, as opposed to men's major stress, which is feeling overwhelmed with responsibility. The women who head corporations, run their own businesses, and generally call the shots are much less stressed than those who sit at a console and answer phones all day or work on an assembly line where they can't even go to the bathroom without asking permission.

If you basically like yourself and admire your accomplishments, your self-esteem and self-confidence can go a long way to combat stress at the office. Knowing you have the power to turn things around can make a big difference when deadlines are tight and supervisors are making demands. The following are a few quick tips to alleviate the tension that comes naturally at the workplace.

## How to Combat Stress on the Job

1. *Get organized.* If you know where things are in the office, on your desk, and in your files, you can work more efficiently.

2. *Avoid misunderstandings.* If you're giving instructions to an employee or receiving them from your superior, spend extra time going over them. This way, you'll avoid misunderstandings. "Would you repeat those instructions back to me so I can be sure we got it straight?" is a perfectly legitimate question for either of you.

3. *Be honest.* If you never lie in your business dealings, you never have to cover up.

4. *Leave a little time between appointments, instead of scheduling them back to back.* You need transition time between one activity and the next. If you're traveling to see a client, allow yourself an additional twenty minutes of travel time, just in case.

5. *Rely on your own self-appreciation more than that of others.* If you get praise for a job, that's great, but it's much less stressful not to anticipate it or to depend on it.

6. *Learn from any criticism you receive.* If your job performance appraisals aren't up to snuff, it's useless and destructive to wallow in negative feelings. Go over your critique carefully to see what you can change so that you'll get a better evaluation the next time around.

7. *Let go of any victim feeling that you're just getting dumped on "because you're a woman."* If you consider your work the equal of everyone else's, hopefully others will too. Feeling sorry for yourself because of your gender, race, religion, or any other category is hardly constructive. Target the problem and fix it.

8. *Accept the fact that you can't have total control.* Working with a team means that there will always be a shifting power structure and other people with competing priorities. That means you probably won't meet every deadline or fill every quota. Just learn to live with it and do what you can to make the team a real support group.

9. *Learn how to say "no" to projects that are nonessential.*

10. *Learn to delegate responsibility to others, just as you do at home.*

11. *Forgive yourself for your mistakes and errors in judgment.* If you can step back and see your errors in a new light, you may open up a wider

range of possibilities. There usually isn't just one right way to do anything—maybe this mistake will lead you to a different and more creative solution.

## CHANGING YOUR BODY AND MIND: BREATHING, SLEEPING AND RELAXATION TECHNIQUES

In order to live longer and better, it's vital to keep changing, and keep adapting to new challenges. Even a mountain changes shape as it's affected over time by weather and water. For a mountain, this takes centuries, but thankfully, it doesn't take that long for people. We can do it with a single decision, or at the most over the course of a few years.

But before you can alter the habits of a lifetime, you have to start with the basics—sleeping, breathing, and relaxing. You think you know how to do all these things already? I ask you, for the sake of good stress management, to start from scratch and pretend you're doing them for the first time.

### Sleep Well and Age Well

Sleep is a healer. As Shakespeare said, it "knits up the ravelled sleave of care." Deprived of sleep for any length of time, we may actually feel that we are going out of our mind. On the other hand, after a restful night, when we relax down to the deepest levels, we may burst out of bed ready to take on the world.

Although most of us need about six to eight hours of sleep a night, some of us can get by on as little as four. There is a goodly number of high-energy individuals who don't require the same respite as others of us. However, everyone needs some time to rest and recover from daily stress.

We are all governed by *circadian cycles*—inner clocks that tick away and allow us to shape the schedules of our lives. The word circadian comes from *circa* meaning *around*, and *dies*, or *day*. During the natural twenty-four-hour cycle, we adjust to dark and light, and work or play within the structure of our time preferences. Our body temperature is at its peak about dusk, when we've finished our daily work, and at its low around 3 or 4 A.M., when we're fast asleep. A dip in energy during the day occurs about 2 P.M., after a full morning's work and a large meal.

We're all quite unique as to our internal clocks. Some of us are larks, able to rise before the sun and get moving immediately while others of us are owls, and only come to life after the sun goes down. It's hard for a woman who's a lark to be married to an owl, and vice versa, since timing in a relationship is so important. If you're ready for bed when your partner is ready to party, stress between you may be the unhappy result.

Some women are susceptible to a decrease in the pattern of available light when seasons change. The doldrums of winter can cause such individuals to suffer from *seasonal affective disorder*, or SAD. The pattern of exposure to light and darkness can drastically affect mood because of changes in the rate of secretion of melatonin. Those who lack sufficient melatonin may also lack sufficient *serotonin*, a neurotransmitter that helps maintain a good mood.

So not only do we need sufficient rest, we also need it at the right time. To alleviate stress, we have to achieve a balance between our inner rhythms and our obligations to the outside world. There's no point in trying to stay up late when your body and brain can't sustain sufficient interest to make it worthwhile.

What can you do to use your sleep time more effectively and simultaneously reduce the stress in your life?

1. *Maintain a regular bedtime.* Your body and mind react favorably to a stable pattern, allowing you to drop off more quickly and to get down to the deeper levels of sleep that are restful and restorative.

2. *Develop a bedtime ritual.* You might want to end your day by reading, or by writing a list of things to do for the next day. Some people find some late-night TV just the soporific to get them to fall asleep easily; others may choose a short period of prayer or meditation to get them relaxed.

3. *Do some form of daily exercise.* There is nothing that will prepare you for a good night's sleep better than a brisk two-mile walk, a half-hour swim, or a daily session of yoga or tai chi chuan. Even sexual activity (either alone or partnered) can be a wonderful relaxer. When

your muscles have really worked hard, it's easier for your body to relax. But don't exercise just before bedtime—it's too stimulating and may rev you up.

4. *Cut out or cut down on caffeine.* Caffeine is a stimulant that causes the heart to pump more quickly. Once carried by the bloodstream up to the brain, it stimulates the cerebral cortex and causes us to feel alert, or even restless and agitated. As our bodies and brains become used to this arousal, we may crave more caffeine in order to recapture that alert feeling.

If you have trouble sleeping, the best advice I can offer is to remove caffeine from your life entirely and stop the cycle before it begins. A cool glass of water or fruit juice will refresh you a lot better than a cup of caffeine. If you can't eliminate it completely, cut down to one or two cups of caffeineated beverages a day. A cup of brewed coffee has about 100 mg.; a twelve-ounce soda, about half that much, and a chocolate bar, about a third as much as that.

To relax before bed, drink a glass of warm milk For added tryptophan, blend in a banana.

5. *Cut out alcohol and sleeping pills.* Alcohol will initially cause you to feel relaxed and sleepy, but will end up disturbing your sleep just several hours later.

Sleeping pills will put you to sleep. But their effect is reduced over time as the brain adapts to them. You may find yourself unable to fall asleep without them. They may affect your waking life as well. Your performance the following day may not be as sharp. A class of sleeping pills known as hypnotics have a cumulative effect—that is, they build up in your system over time, significantly altering your brain and body function.

6. *Sleep in a cool room.* Your body temperature decreases at night because your metabolism slows down. As long as you have enough blankets or a comforter to retain your body heat, you might want to try opening a window to ensure there is good circulation and sufficient oxygen in your room.

7. *If you can't fall asleep, get up and do something relaxing.* Tossing and turning can be very stressful. All those hours wasted lying in bed staring at the ceiling, going over problems you've been dealing with all day. So make good use of your time—get up and read, listen to music, write some letters. Don't do anything overly stimulating

though, such as balancing your checkbook or planning your work day. After an hour or so, you can lie down and try again.

## Taking in the Breath of Life

It may amaze you to learn that it's possible you don't know the best way to breathe. You used to know as a baby, but you've possibly forgotten. Life's stresses might have made you stop breathing from your belly and start breathing with your chest and shoulders. You take only shallow inhalations, and occasionally feel short of breath.

For better health management, you owe it to yourself to breathe deeply and completely. This means that you'll have to spend some time becoming aware of how you breathe now and changing your pattern over time. It will feel uncomfortable at first, but after a while, it'll seem as if you've been breathing this way all your life.

## How to Breathe

1. Stand in front of a mirror and breathe in whatever way feels natural to you. Watch the rise and fall of your chest and shoulders, and try not to strain in any way as you inhale and exhale.

2. This exercise is particularly difficult for those women who are typically self-conscious about their stomachs. But it's necessary if they want to live longer and look younger. I want you to put both hands on your belly, about three inches above your waist. Inhale and let your stomach push your hands out from your abdomen with your breath. Next, exhale and allow your hands to get sucked in by your belly.

3. Think of your inhalation and exhalation as one flowing movement. Be sure to give yourself sufficient time to take in as much air as you want. If you feel at all lightheaded, sit down and return to the breathing pattern that feels comfortable to you. Try this new one again tomorrow.

4. Whenever you're in the midst of a difficult situation, or you feel particularly stressed, stop what you're doing and concentrate on breathing. Not only will it make you focus on something other than your problem, but it will also allow you to take in more oxygen. This in turn will help you think more clearly.

5. As you lie in bed at night, and your body is settling, take a few deep breaths into your abdomen to help alleviate the tensions that may have built up over the course of the day. If you're having trouble falling asleep, your body will relax more as you learn this healthful method of breathing. And when you do drop off, you will sleep better too.

## Relaxation: A Daily Practice

There is a marked difference between "zoning out" in front of a TV and relaxing. In a laboratory, when television viewers were hooked up to an electroencephalograph, which measures brain waves, it was found that the subjects were neither alert nor aware, but rather, half asleep.

Meditators, on the other hand, who may appear to be in a trance, are actually concentrating. What is meditation? A learned, practiced method of tuning into your awareness and allowing yourself to eliminate outside distractions. Studies have shown that insomniacs, after having practiced a particular form of meditation for thirty days, could reduce the time they required to fall asleep from a norm of 75 minutes to just 15 minutes. The reason, of course, is that meditation teaches us to concentrate effectively. It also gives us control of many bodily functions previously thought to be involuntary.

Meditation, which involves sitting quietly and clearing your mind of extraneous thoughts, is wonderful at stress reduction, although you may have to work at getting used to it. There are a number of structured techniques that you can employ in your own stress management program. Here are some you can try.

1. *Meditation.* Although meditation is a centuries-old practice, it was first studied as a tool for stress management in the late 1960s by Herbert Benson, a researcher at Harvard Medical School. Benson discovered that daily meditators with several years' practice evoked what he called "the relaxation response." During meditation blood pressure was lowered, heart rate slowed and muscle tension decreased. He also found that the participants in his study needed less oxygen during meditation and that practitioners could lower their oxygen consumption rates in minutes—something that ordinarily takes hours of sleep to accomplish.

Some meditators concentrate on their breath, others on one word, such as *calm* or *peace* or *one*. Still others attempt to watch each thought passing through their mind as though they were on a moving train and their thoughts were the scenery. The idea is not to hold onto anything, but just to let yourself be witness to it.

"Mindfulness meditation," where you focus your attention on whatever you are currently doing, be it writing your signature or concentrating on your beloved's face is often a good way to ease into meditation for beginners. After learning to stay in the present moment during your routine, everyday activities, it becomes easier to do the same during sitting meditation.

Meditation is an ancient practice. A devoted American follower of an Indian guru brought meditation to America, and during the 1970s, nearly a million practitioners emulated the Beatles' new attraction to this pursuit. Meditation can be done sitting and relaxing with your eyes closed on your own for ten to twenty minutes a day. There is ritual involved in this type of practice as well—you can burn incense and, at the beginning and end of each session ring a bell or gong.

A nursing home study designed to see whether meditation could prolong life had remarkable results. Seventy-three residents of different retirement homes, with an average age of 81 years, were randomly assigned to three groups. One group was given no instructions about relaxing; one group was taught various relaxation techniques, and one was taught meditation.

At the end of three years, over one third of the first group had died, $12^1/_2$ percent of the relaxation group had died, yet every member of the meditation group was still going strong.

You don't have to sit to meditate. If you engage in some activity in a thoughtful, focused manner, thinking of nothing but that activity, you can achieve a similar result. Gardening, rock climbing, or lap swimming are just three pursuits that offer an opportunity to get yourself into a meditative state.

2. *Visualization.* This technique allows you to create a picture in your mind in order to accomplish a goal. If your stomach is in knots at the end of a stressful day, you can visualize yourself untying the knots and smoothing them out flat. If you get tension headaches, you

might picture your unwanted headache as a concrete block that you can put into a box, wrap with Scotch tape and paper, and pull right out of your head.

3. *Yoga*. This is the ancient Indian practice of placing your body in various postures or *asanas* and holding them as you breathe deeply into them. The benefits to mind and body have been acknowledged by the medical community. For instance, Dr. Dean Ornish of the Preventive Medicine Research Institute in San Francisco feels that yoga is an essential part of any stress management program and has been able to persuade several insurance companies to reimburse participants in his reversal of heart disease program for their yoga practice. Yoga enables people to keep the energy of mind and body in balance. (See the yoga exercises on p. 119.)

4. *Tai chi chuan*. This ancient Chinese meditative art offers the discipline of moving postures, slow choreographed routines or "forms," that activate mind and body. Daily *tai chi* practice gives the body strength, endurance and flexibility, lowers blood pressure, and calms the mind. It incorporates the principles of *yin* and *yang*, one black and one white tear-shaped drop interlocked within a circle, each with a dot of the other color inside it. This icon is the perfect representation for balance; when we are less stressed, we accept that our dark side and our light side are both intrinsic parts of us.

5. *Biofeedback*. This technique uses monitoring equipment in an office or laboratory. You can be taught by a trainer to alter involuntary bodily functions such as blood pressure, temperature and heart rate by attending to audio or visual feedback (flashing lights, for example) from a machine. After several sessions with a trainer, you are able to take these techniques home with you and alter your own stress patterns.

6. *Self-hypnosis*. It is possible to take yourself to a level of deep relaxation and give yourself suggestions that will alleviate stress. You may be able to visualize your tense muscles as flowers, opening and expanding in the sunlight. The power of this suggestion may allow you to actually smell a floral aroma and feel the warmth of the sun as you concentrate. Through relaxation and self-suggestion to control sensory input, you can successfully learn to manage stress.

7. *Prayer*. Prayer can be as helpful as meditation, and may be the preference of those of you who come from a religious tradition. Not

only can you center yourself and clear your mind of extraneous thoughts, you also have a foundation, a belief in something greater than yourself. Prayer can thus reduce the pressures of your life and help you to relax.

## Creating a Relaxation Environment

Whatever form of practice you choose, you need the proper surroundings in order to forget your daily stress and take your mind off your problems.

1. Select a comfortable, cool, quiet spot with soft lighting. You may sit cross-legged on a mat or cushion on the floor, or in a straight-backed chair. It's not advisable to lie down, because you might fall asleep. The idea of meditation is to become more rather than less aware.

2. Spend a few moments allowing the last busy thoughts of your day to pass through your mind. Relax your eyes, but don't close them. Just get in the mood to relax.

3. Now close your eyes. Concentrate either on your breath or on a word of your choice. You may want to count downward slowly from one hundred to zero by ten. As you count backward, feel the decades slipping off you. You will actually feel your age slowing down along with your heart rate and respiration.

4. You may find that you aren't able to stay with the counting or single word throughout your first meditation. If you feel your mind "chattering" away, listen to the disrupting thoughts and then let them go. It's perfectly normal to feel drawn back into your habitual patterns of thinking; don't blame yourself but allow yourself gradually to get back on track.

5. Don't set any goals. This in itself is your reward. You don't have to have a great revelation, or feel as if your backache or headache has vanished. All you have to do is just be there.

6. If you find yourself drifting in and out of consciousness, try to pull your mind back to your breathing. You are aiming to stay alert, and concentrating on a physical process will help you do that.

7. Enjoy the quiet moments as you experience them, one at a time. You may find, as you continue your practice, that there are times when you feel blocked and other times when there is a flow of energy. Each meditation is different. Just be open to each one.

# NINE STEPS TO ANTIAGING STRESS MANAGEMENT

If you take a fresh perspective to your stresses you'll be able to handle them better. We all tend to repeat our patterns of worrying over and over, whether or not they work. Sometimes, our old coping mechanisms just create more work and anxiety.

When we take a stand against our problems, we in fact give ourselves a needed boost of energy—and longevity. Following the nine steps below, you will see your difficulties changing shape and becoming more manageable. Consequently, you will feel less burdened, more competent, and more receptive to enjoying life.

## 1. Manage Your Time, and Prioritize Your Tasks

What's so important that it has to be done immediately? What's important but can wait until tomorrow? What's relatively insignificant, a task that need only get done when you have an extra hour or two to spare?

Sit down and draw up a list in which you define the various challenges you face on a daily, weekly, monthly, and annual basis. Then draw a line through out the ones you can learn to live without. You need to list everything, from first priorities such as health and fitness, money management, career development, and personal relationships, to a second tier of concerns, such as home improvement, going back to school, or saving enough money to travel or retire from the job you're currently doing. (You'll never want to quit doing at least some form of work, since having something important to do each day prolongs life.)

Give yourself credit for everything you've accomplished to date, and consider what you've learned from past experience. Then look ahead and see where you'd like to be five years from now, ten years from now, or twenty years from now.

## 2. Manage Your Roles

How many people are you? If you are wife, mother, child, lover, employee, employer, chief cook and bottlewasher, comedian, psychotherapist, financial analyst, janitor, chauffeur, and so on, it's time to put a limit to the number of hats you think you must wear. No one, not even Superwoman, can possibly do all these jobs simultaneously and do them well.

Just as you prioritize and manage your time, you must manage your roles. There will be some you love to shoulder, and even if they cause you stress, they're the kind you enjoy. You welcome the challenges and meet them with open arms. There are other roles in which you probably procrastinate and don't perform very well. If they're giving you too much distress, how about negotiating with your partner, children, or friends to take them on for you, at least some of the time? Of course, if you decide to give up some of these roles, you'll have to dredge up the strength and motivation to ask others to help.

No woman is an island, and many hands make light work. Rather than brave it alone, enlist your friends and family to assist you. If people ask you for favors, ask them to reciprocate in kind. If you can't reach people when you first try them, don't give up and assume they won't help. Be persuasive (not nagging), and you'll find you have a battery of assistants at your disposal. The job may not get done exactly as you would do it, but you may be astounded at how well—and how differently—it can be done by someone else.

## 3. Form a Support Group

A real stress-reduction technique is to set up a support group among friends, a kind of extended family where everyone helps everyone else. It's been shown that support groups preserve life—Dr. David Spiegel's studies on breaking social isolation, for instance, are positive examples of how becoming part of a group can extend life. The women in his breast cancer survivor groups who met regularly after their surgery while they were undergoing chemotherapy or radiation,

As you become more aware of your own emotional balance, it will be easier for you to deal with your partner, your children and your parents. They won't always do everything the way you want them to—so give up trying to fit them into your mold. Just as you give yourself room to stretch and change, be sure to give them the same opportunity. And remember to laugh when you can!

If you're upset with your child, for example, sit back before you criticize and try to see his or her perspective. You may find the behavior a demand for more attention. Don't blame yourself for being unable to see this till now—the ability to empathize is not inborn, but comes to us slowly over time. It needs to be developed, nurtured, and thoughtfully maintained. As you deal with your child in this new way, it may seem at first as though you're giving in. Instead, think of it as yielding—giving a little from your own core of strength to add to that of your child. This way, you'll feel much more helpful, much less put-upon. Learn from your children how to be a better parent in a sharing process. And over the long haul, it can result in a great deal of emotional balance both for you and for them.

## 8. Deal with Your Past and Future to Make the Present Better

The person you are today is molded by the child you once were, the adolescent you became, the adult you are now, and the person you hope to be someday.

If you had a difficult childhood, including perhaps abuse or trauma, you will have additional work to do on stress management. Instead of blaming others, feeling sorry for yourself and carrying your depression into the present, take a positive approach. The past is over and done with; you can't correct it or change it, but you can certainly learn from it. There's formal learning, the kind that ends with a certificate from an educational institution, and there's the kind we get from the school of life. Think how wise you are, to have gathered all this experience. It's all useful.

Detach yourself from the past for a moment and answer the following questions: How did you overcome your trauma? How did this challenge make you a stronger and more sympathetic individual? What can you teach others because of your knowledge? How can you pass your strength of character on to your children? How can you forgive your parents, or those who hurt you, so that you can go on with your life? No matter what they did or who they were, they too have human qualities and human dilemmas that can help you to understand your own. And *those* are the elements that you can pass on to the next generation. Those are the elements that can help you to heal yourself.

Use the past well and wisely, and it can help you not only today, but each subsequent day of your life.

## 9. Allow Yourself a Few Failures

Nobody's perfect—not even you! It would be quite dull if you did everything right all the time. Children learn after touching a hot stove not to do it again; we can also learn from the emotional blips and glitches that occur in adulthood. Only by looking at our inappropriate choices can we ever hope to learn "wrong" from "right," and how to change our behavior.

## What You Can Do to Stop Worrying

Worrying doesn't solve anything—it simply grows on itself in a spiral of increasing worry. One anxious thought breeds the next, and out of it emerges an even bigger range of negativity. If you're caught up in feeling bad, you may actually forget why you started to worry in the first place. Yet you feel trapped, with no way out.

No, you can't easily brainwash yourself and simply erase negative thoughts from your mind. You can, however, make a real difference in the quality of your stress by actively working on a problem instead of sitting and mulling over it ad nauseum. Here *are* some useful approaches to worrying:

1. *Pick a worry time and stick to it.* A little worry, like an occasional piece of chocolate cake in a diet, is manageable. Worrying all the time is destructive and time-consuming. So instead of worrying at random, in an uncontrolled manner, discipline yourself to worry at special set times. You can take one half-hour a day—a good time might be midway through the day, or maybe at 5:30, during your transition from work to home. Do all your worrying then, and any other time you feel like worrying, remind yourself, "I'll just have to deal with that at 5:30" and put it out of your mind until then.

You can also assign one half-day a week for problem solving. I allot Friday mornings to doing what I can to take care of my worries, and you can do the same. Call people who might have a direct bearing on what's bothering you, either because they're directly involved, or because they have some expertise or a special contact with someone who can help. Don't gripe—just get the problem out in the open, offer a few ideas of your own and ask for their suggestions. If you discover that no one can help you, at least you know you're on your own and can begin to research other options.

2. *Attack your worries rationally.* If you identify the problem, you can more easily attack it directly. You don't have to worry about all its possible shades and meanings; all you have to do is meet the problem head-on. It's sometimes a good idea to use a friend or family member as a sounding board so that you can evaluate the best options together. Again, try to keep a balance between feelings and reason. The more dispassionately you can look at your problems, the more likely you are to arrive at a rational solution.

3. *Take a proactive approach.* Don't wait for problems to come to you. Instead of simply reacting out of weakness and vulnerability, decide clearly on a course of action and act assertively. You can go after what you want. Having a goal is exciting and gives you something to work toward. When you know what you want, you can do the opposite of worrying—you can visualize your success. This in turn will encourage you to start considering the small steps you have to take in order to get to your eventual destination. Whether your proactive plan has to do with finance, romance, or longevity, you can get there best if you travel in one determined direction.

4. *Visualize Success.* The writer Shakti Gawain urges us to take charge of our lives with "creative visualization," a technique whereby we create in our minds the reality we wish to attain. By painting a detailed picture of your goals, you're able to mentally rehearse those steps necessary for success. If your attitude is a winning one, you'll be hard to defeat.

## Stress Is Just Another Word for Progress

The more you see yourself as capable of success, the less you'll tend to worry. Of course, the road may be bumpy, the obstacles many, but with the desire to keep going, your motivation is assured. And the desire to attain success, stressful as it may be, is the reason you took the road in the first place. Relax and enjoy your journey, one day at a time, moment by moment.

## Yoga Exercises to Lengthen Your Life

I've found that yoga is an easy, comfortable stress manager that takes very little time and can be done virtually anywhere with no necessary equipment except for a carpeted floor.

The yoga postures or *asanas* restore youthful flexibility and allow body and mind to come into harmony. Remember to build your flexibility for these positions slowly, particularly if you haven't done any stretching exercises for a while. Never strain or push yourself, and wait about two hours after eating to begin your practice. Wear loose clothing, remove your shoes, and breathe deeply.

1. *Knee to head.* Lying with your back flat on the floor, bring one leg up, bending at the knee. With your hands on your calf, pull your knee gently toward your body. Now pull your head up to reach for your knee. Alternate with your other leg and repeat five times on each side.

2. *The frog.* Sit on the floor with the soles of your feet together and your knees spread apart. Grab your ankles and push your elbows into your knees, curling your head to your chest and then pulling down toward your ankles. Do five repetitions.

3. *The cobra.* Lie on your stomach with your legs and feet together. Place your palms under your shoulders with your fingertips just extending beyond your shoulders. Looking up toward the ceiling, raise your chest off the floor using your back muscles, not your arms. Now arch your back even more, pressing your belly button into the floor. Breathe into this pose and hold it for ten to twenty seconds. Then slowly return to the floor, turning your face to one side. Turn your hands over, palms up, and relax for twenty seconds before repeating the pose. Do five repetitions.

4. *The locust.* Lie on your stomach with your arms outstretched to the sides, your palms down, legs together. Raise your eyes toward the ceiling, raise your chest off the floor, then lift your arms and legs off

the floor. Enjoy this "flying" posture for ten seconds as you breathe and balance on the center of your abdomen. Keep your legs and knees together. Come down slowly, turn your head to one side, turn your palms up and relax for twenty seconds. Repeat five times. At first you should hold this posture for no more than five seconds, then build up to ten.

5. *The half-moon.* Standing with your feet together, raise your arms over your head, palms together, thumbs crossed and locked. Keep your head up and your chin forward. With your arms tight against your ears, stretch for the sky.

Now slowly bend your arms and body backward as far as you can go without strain, keeping your arms straight and breathing into the posture. Focus your attention on the back of your neck and relax into the arch.

· Return slowly to center, then reach straight upward. Now bend forward at the waist and grab your lower calves, and attempt to bring your forehead toward your knees. Hold this pose for five seconds at first and build up to ten.

Return slowly to center and lower your arms. Do this exercise only once per day for the first week, then add a second repetition during your second week.

6. *The soaring eagle.* Stand naturally, feet together, and then move your right foot out about four feet so that you are standing in a straddle position. Raise both arms to the side, parallel to the floor, your palms facing downward. Keep your knees straight but not locked. Now bend forward at the waist and grab the backs of your ankles, fingers together and thumbs on the outsides of your feet. Bring your head toward your legs by allowing your upper body to sink. Breathe into this posture and see if each breath will take you even lower. Think about lifting your "sitting bones" up to the ceiling. Come back to standing and repeat this posture five times.

7. *The relaxer.* This one seems easy, but for some tense individuals, it's the toughest. Lie on your back, arms comfortably at your sides, palms facing upward, with your legs comfortably apart. Close your eyes and let go of as much tension as you can release. Imagine yourself as heavy as a piece of lead, fully supported and able to sink even deeper into the floor. Enjoy this relaxed, "heavy" sensation.

If you can apply yourself to practicing these postures every day for two months, you'll begin to feel a definite sense of renewed youth and vigor. Your body will be freer of tension, much more limber and generally healthier. You'll feel more balanced in mind, body and spirit. And you will have given yourself a precious gift to enjoy for the rest of your life.

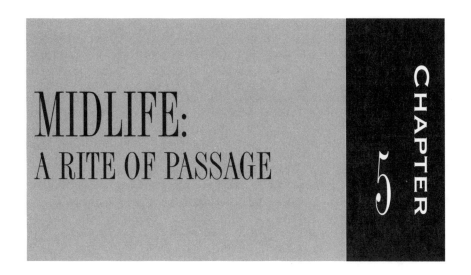

# MIDLIFE:
## A RITE OF PASSAGE

CHAPTER 5

$T$he question, said a wise woman, is not how old you are, but *how* you are old. If we think about midlife as the jumping off place for what we do with the second fifty years we've been granted, it becomes really exciting—especially since women in midlife today can choose their own adventures.

This generation of baby-boomers is taking over, quite literally, because there are so many of them. The group of women born right after World War II is at the forefront of the changing demographics of America. By the year 2016, there will be more women in our country over the age of menopause than under it. If we look at pictures of our grandmothers at 50, they seem elderly, tired, finished with what they considered the useful (read, "reproductive") part of their lives. How different for women today, who at 50 are just making inroads into the second half of life.

The lifespan of women has increased dramatically, from about 47 at the turn of the century (when many women died in childbirth or from septic conditions in the hospitals where they delivered) to approximately 78 today. There are many active, vital women in their 80s and 90s who have grown up instead of grown old, model examples of the wisdom and maturity that comes with additional years.

Unfortunately, society's image of the older woman has not quite caught up with reality, and we are still handicapped by a lack of pos-

123

itive role models in print ads, film, and TV. It is therefore a challenge to all women in midlife to forge their own unique roles for the future and to improve their self-image as they celebrate each successive birthday.

## MENOPAUSE: A PHYSICAL, MENTAL, EMOTIONAL, AND SPIRITUAL CHANGE

Menopause (from the Latin *meno* meaning "month" and *pausus* meaning "cessation") literally means the end of menstruation. It is that moment in time when your monthly cycle stops for good. This can be a point of joyous celebration for many—no more cramps or worry about becoming pregnant. Most women may have a period one month, then notice subtle changes in their cycle, then a little spotting, and then they may actually forget to keep track. Most experts consider you past menopause if two years have gone by without any bleeding.

This change of hormonal status generally occurs between your forty-fifth and fifty-fifth birthdays, though the range can be even larger. Statistically, the average age of occurrence is 51 years and 4 months, but many life events can alter this number. Being a heavy smoker brings on early menopause. The telling event is how soon you begin to experience a rapid decline in production of the gonadal hormone, *estrogen*. This hormone, with its companion, *progesterone*, keeps the menstrual cycle going and also affects the brain, heart, and bones.

The period of time during which your periods may become irregular and finally slow to a halt as ovulation ceases is known as the *climacteric*. This is a Greek word, referring to the steps of a ladder. The Greeks saw life as divided into seven-year segments, and the time from 42 to 63 was an individual's chance to climb to the top rung of the ladder. If we think about midlife as rising to the top, we can forever do away with such offensive expressions as "over the hill." To the Greeks, getting older meant becoming more mature, more sophisticated, and better able to counsel others still too young to know their own minds and hearts.

Let's get the terminology straight. If your periods are becoming irregular but you still menstruate, you are in *premenopause*. During those years when you begin to experience hot flashes, vaginal dryness or other signs and signals of change, you are in *peri-menopause*. If you no longer bleed, you have passed *menopause*. After this time, you are *post-menopausal*.

## THE FEMALE LIFE CYCLE

Women are born with about a million eggs in each of their two ovaries, and that's as many as they'll ever produce. By the time they reach puberty, many of these fledgling eggs have dissolved into the tissue of the ovary, and only about 500,000 remain. By the time they hit menopause, most women have about 300 or 400 eggs left, which are generally not viable in terms of fertilization.

If we think about the female life cycle, there are roughly three periods after childhood. The first, when hormonal production begins, is *puberty*. The second, when women produce eggs in their ovaries that can be fertilized and can bear children, is known as the *reproductive stage*. The third, as hormonal production declines and women become anovulatory, is *postmenopause*.

Hormones are chemical messengers that travel through the body to reach and stimulate a particular target organ. In the case of our gonadal or sex hormones, these have a lot of influence over what makes us tick—what makes us the particular people we are. This stimulation, of course, is not just physical. Because the mind and body are so intimately related, a great deal of what we think and feel as men or women can be determined by where we are in the life cycle.

### Your Menstrual Cycle

When you first started to menstruate, you may remember bouts of crying and depression alternating with feelings of wonder, elation, or downright silliness. You were worried about the zits suddenly springing out on your face, about whether you might start spotting when you were wearing your new white skirt, and whether anybody (male or female) would ever call you. A similar feeling of being on an emotional rollercoaster happens to women when they first become pregnant, and then happens again just before they hit menopause.

In order to understand this hormonal turbulence, we have to go back to the first big change, from childhood to puberty. For about a year before your menses begins, your brain is getting ready to help the body facilitate this process. What happens is this: The master gland, the *hypothalamus*, produces a hormone called GnRH which in turn triggers the *pituitary* gland to start secreting two hormones that target the endocrine system. FSH (follicle stimulating hormone) is produced at the beginning of your monthly cycle, and LH (luteinizing hormone) in the middle of the cycle.

FSH tells the ovaries to start producing *estrogen*, which encourages the development of several different eggs, one of which will mature sufficiently to ovulate. As the egg ripens, the pituitary starts cutting back on FSH and starts putting out LH, which causes the follicle to release the egg in the process called *ovulation*. After the follicle lets go of the egg, it begins to produce *progesterone*, the hormone responsible for creating a nourishing environment in which the egg can grow. Then the egg continues its passage down the fallopian tube toward the uterus.

When this happens, the brain cuts back on its FSH and LH production, which in turn, stops the flow of estrogen and progesterone. With no hormonal stimulation to supply a rich blood source for the lining of the uterus, the *endometrium*, it detaches and thus discharge is expelled. This process happens month after month, year after year, unless you become pregnant, or undergo surgery to have your ovaries removed.

As you reach menopause, however, the brain-endocrine signals get fuzzy. As fewer and fewer viable eggs exist less estrogen is produced, the brain frantically tries to balance the system by making more FSH. More and more cycles are *anovulatory*, where there isn't sufficient hormonal stimulation to ripen an egg but there is still enough to allow some tissue to release from the uterine lining. You may spot or stain for a few days and then several weeks later, you may bleed profusely as more of the endometrium comes free. At last, when you are producing perhaps a fifth of the amount of estrogen you had during your reproductive years, your periods stop entirely. (Your body will still continue to produce a weaker form of estrogen known as *estrone*, which is produced by your ovaries and adrenal glands.)

With the loss of abundant estrogen, many different organs and tissues begin to undergo some significant changes. But if you keep in mind that your body will return to homeostasis within a few years when it adjusts to its new hormonal environment, none of these menopausal changes should really be overwhelming. Remember that these too shall pass.

## THE SIGNS AND SIGNALS OF MENOPAUSE

Whenever I hear about someone who's gone to her doctor with menopausal "symptoms," I want to stop and inform her that symptoms only come with disease, and menopause is no such thing. The various psychobiological and chemical changes that occur in all women are only partly due to menopause—everything else is due to the aging process, which begins the moment we're born. So the sooner we can think about menopause as a stage of life the sooner we can adjust to the changes that do occur.

Estrogen, as I mentioned before, affects the body as an entire system. The way that a drop in estrogen alters the heart and bones is far more crucial than any other changes that occur, such as hot flashes, vaginal dryness, insomnia, or changes in the breasts and skin.

1. *The heart.* One reason that most women don't succumb to heart attacks in their early forties as men do is that they are protected by their high levels of estrogen. One of the jobs of this hormone is to keep blood lipid levels balanced, maximizing the *high-density lipoproteins* (HDLs) and minimizing the *low-density lipoproteins* (LDLs). It's that particular mix of "good" and "bad" cholesterol that you have to worry about when estrogen levels drop after menopause. Another beneficial effect of estrogen is that it keeps the blood vessels elastic, allowing good circulation to all bodily organs and tissues. This property, too, is greatly diminished after menopause as estrogen levels drop.

### What to Do to Protect Your Heart

See Chapter Two for a good midlife diet and Chapter Nine to learn what to do to prevent heart disease.

☐ Make sure you have regular, daily exercise which helps keep your HDLs high.

☐ Engage in a regular program of stress reduction.

☐ See later sections in this chapter on hormone replacement therapy and alternative treatments.

2. *The bones*. We have two types of bone: the hard, shiny white bone (*cortical* bone) on the outside, and the inner *trabecular* bone, an interlocking network of minerals, blood vessels, and marrow that holds the structure together. Estrogen helps to keep the calcium in our bones as opposed to letting it leach out into the blood stream. But after menopause, both the mass and density of bone decrease at a rate of about one to two percent a year for typical midlife women, and a rate of five to six percent a year for rapid bone losers. These are the women who are in most danger of hip fractures and vertebral breaks after menopause. Since a woman's bone structure is generally smaller and thinner than a man's, she is at greater risk of contracting osteoporosis (literal meaning: "porous bones") as she loses estrogen.

## What to Do to Protect Your Bones:

☐ Follow a program of regular weight-bearing exercises, such as walking, jogging, dancing, aerobics, or martial arts.

☐ Make sure you take at least 1,000 mg. of calcium before menopause and 1,200 after, combined with half as much magnesium.

☐ Have a bone densitometry test to see whether you are a standard or rapid bone loser and to make a determination with your physician as to whether you might be a good candidate for hormone replacement therapy (refer to discussion on p. 136 of this chapter).

☐ Have your eyes checked to see if you need glasses. Safety-proof your house against loose wires and rugs on which you can trip.

See Chapter Seven for a full discussion of osteoporosis, including simple exercises and back-saver tips.

3. *Hot flashes and night sweats.* The most common sign of menopause in the Western world, reported by 40 percent to 88 percent of women surveyed, (depending on which study you read), is the hot flash. Hot flashes seem to be acknowledged by certain cultures and not others; studies in Japan, Mexico, Pakistan, and Hong Kong estimate that only 10 percent of women suffer from them. Although we're not sure why this is so, part of it apparently has to do with differences in diet (these countries consume high levels of phytoestrogens in their foods) and much of it may have to do with a more positive attitude toward older women.

But in our country, the hot flash is a very common occurrence. You may be in the midst of a meeting at work, sitting in a restaurant, taking a jog on the beach, when suddenly you can be overwhelmed with the shock of intense heat often accompanied by an accelerated heartbeat. Your face and chest may turn beet red. Then, about three to four minutes later, you may be shaking with chills as your body attempts to compensate for the rapid rise and fall in temperature.

One woman aptly described this experience to me as feeling "like a boiled tomato with the skin ready to burst." Many women think they've come down with the flu when they have their first hot flash. These flashes may occur as often as seven times per hour, or may happen to you once a month. Typically, they are more frequent and intense at the onset of your climacteric, and over the next few years, they taper off.

What's really going on is that your hypothalamus, functioning as the thermometer in your body, is confused by your shifting hormonal responses. When your estrogen levels start dropping, the brain attempts to bump up production by sending more urgent messages of its own. Instead of putting out a continuous amount of hormone to stimulate the pituitary, the hypothalamus begins reacting with other releasing hormones. Researchers feel that this action causes the body to respond as though it's overheated.

Flashes seem to occur at certain particular hours for most women, and many experience them when they're sleeping—thus the term, "night sweats." Naturally, if you are wakened frequently during the night and are soaking wet, it's difficult to get back to those restorative deeper levels of sleep. You may recall how wooly-headed you felt when you had an infant waking you at all hours and you got up in the morning more tired than when you went to bed. The same

better because they no longer have to be concerned with contraception or bleeding or a child rushing in in the midst of a wonderful erotic experience.

## How to Handle Vaginal Dryness

❒ Engage in sex on a regular basis if at all possible. As with any other muscle, you have to use it or you lose it. Results of the Stanford Menopause Study indicate that weekly sex can significantly decrease both the frequency and severity of hot flashes, since sexually active women tend to maintain higher levels of estrogen later in life.

❒ Use a water-based lubricant such as KY Jelly, Replens, Astroglide, or Gyne-Moistrin.

❒ Learn to masturbate and experiment with a vibrator. By teaching yourself what you enjoy in bed without having the pressure of pleasing a partner, you can become more comfortable sexually. Studies have shown that regular masturbation slows down the thinning of the vaginal walls and that weekly sexual activity (whether alone or partnered) may keep the lubrication process active.

See Chapter Six for a discussion of libido and sex drive as you age.

5. *Urinary distress.* Estrogen helps to keep the urinary system functional by nourishing the tissues at the bottom of the pelvic area. Since the bladder lies right next to the uterus, if tumors grow and distend, it may become more difficult to retain urine as you age. Sometimes, just sneezing or coughing or enjoying an orgasm can cause "stress incontinence," or involuntary leaking of urine. The television ads, informing mature women that "protective pads" are likely to be part of their future, are totally misleading. You are not doomed to wearing diapers as you get older!

By practicing Kegel exercises, you can keep your *pubococcygeal muscles* (between your vagina and anus) strong well into your eighties and nineties. To do a Kegel exercise, pretend that you are sitting on the toilet, about to release the flow of urine. Then, contract the muscles as if you are stopping the flow. You will feel your anal sphincter tighten along with the muscles around your vagina. Practice these daily, ten reps at a time, three times a day, and you will not only preserve your urinary health, you will also increase sexual pleasure for yourself and your partner.

There are also behavior modification programs for incontinence that work brilliantly. These involve drinking quantities of liquids and practicing Kegel exercises for increasing periods of time. Ask your health-care provider if you need a referral to begin such a program.

Some women develop urinary incontinence because of a lack of collagen in the pelvic supportive tissues around the urethra. Previously, only surgery could repair a weakened pelvic floor. However, researchers at the University of Southern California School of Medicine are using a new procedure involving collagen injections that seems to have a lot of promise. In this procedure, collagen is injected into the tissue surrounding the urethra, adding bulk and increasing pressure, which helps to minimize urine leakage.

6. *The skin.* As we get older, no matter our gender, we wrinkle. This is because we have less collagen in the skin to retain structure and strength. It's estrogen that keeps collagen under the skin surface, which is the reason that it becomes more difficult in later life to retain that youthful "glow." The layer of fat cells under the skin also declines with age, which is why the skin of older people tends to look thin and drawn.

If you were a sun worshipper in your early years, you can expect to start wrinkling sooner. Exposure to sunlight is responsible for ninety percent of the photoaging process. As we get older, in addition to losing the estrogen that keeps the skin elastic, we also lose our tanning pigments (*melanocytes*), which makes us more susceptible to aging and skin cancer. Heed well my advice on sunproofing your skin in Chapter Eight.

Another experience common to some midlife women is *formication.* This feeling, not quite itching, not quite dryness, can be terribly annoying, but generally a bath with baking soda will alleviate the unpleasantness. Like many other signs of menopause, it tapers off and ceases once the body is in better hormonal balance.

## Additional Changes You Might Encounter at Menopause

The list of possible signs and signals of menopause is too large to print here—from crying jags and dry eyes to thinning hair and mysterious bruises to increased flatulence and weight gain. Some of these changes are part of the aging process, some are hormonal, and some may be unique to your mind and body at this stage of your life. Understand that although these phenomena may be unsettling and uncomfortable, none of them are life-threatening. They are just a part of the midlife journey and should be dealt with as they occur.

7. *Joint pain.* Bursitis in the shoulder, tennis elbow, trick knees, sore ankles, and cramping of various extremities may be related to menopause. Joint aches can be linked to the adrenal glands; this is where the body makes cortisone, which allows the joints to move freely. Since these discomforts are common in both men and women as we age, it's a good idea to have your doctor check them out to determine their source. If they're menopausal, they'll pass pretty quickly; if not, you may need to be referred to an orthopedist or physical therapist.

8. *Migraines.* Migraines are headaches that occur primarily on one side of the brain, and begin with a spasm in an artery close to the surface of the scalp. It is thought that the imbalance in the ratio of estrogen to progesterone or low progesterone levels has something to do with this phenomenon. Migraines may be accompanied by nausea, dizziness, and sensitivity to light. Since we are often alerted to a coming migraine by an aura or sense that something is about to happen, it's possible to try to head one off with breathing and meditation. Some women swear by orgasm as a means of stopping a migraine by producing beta endorphins (those natural opiates in the brain that reduce pain) and directing blood flow from the head to the genitalia.

9. *Tinnitus (ringing in the ears).* This sensory disturbance may respond well to meditation, or to listening to tapes of natural sounds such as waves and wind.

10. *Burning, dry mouth.* Caffeine and antihistamines can aggravate the problem. Although very little is known about this condition, some women find relief in sucking on ice cubes and massaging their gums.

11. *Forgetfulness.* It can be frightening to forget names and words for common everyday items, but it happens. Panic only makes it

worse, and understanding that your neurochemistry is in flux may alleviate some of your fears. A lack of sleep is also sometimes responsible for memory loss, so taking care of your night sweats and insomnia may make your mind clearer. It can be helpful to do mental exercises, make up mnemonic devices, or play memory games in order to work those brain cells. This problem generally dissipates by the end of the climacteric.

12. *Cold extremities.* In order to  warm your hands and feet, you can do visualizations where you imagine holding warm objects, or you can try inverted positions—bend over at your waist, keeping your knees lightly bent, and let your arms dangle in front of you. You should also check your jewelry—make sure your rings, bracelets, and so forth haven't gotten too tight and aren't cutting off circulation.

13. *Auras (prior to a flash).* An aura is a warning before something happens. You may see spots before your eyes and then a gleaming outline of a form; you may feel dizzy, numbness or tingling sensations; you may feel terribly restless. There is nothing other-worldly about an aura—it is simply a signal in the brain that a physical event is about to take place. The good thing about having auras is that you have notification of a flash coming and can quickly drink a glass of water or do some deep breathing—which can often head off the flash!

14. *Shortness of breath and tachycardia (pounding heart).* These two symptoms usually come together, often during a flash. The rise in body temperature can accompany increased heart rate and respiration, and awareness of the event may make you feel anxious and unable to breathe. The best treatment is to sit down and do some deep breathing, quieting your mind by reciting "one" or "calm" and reassuring yourself that the experience will soon be over.

15. *Insomnia.* An inability to sleep may be due to night sweats, but also stems from neurotransmitter imbalances. Also, midlife women may not need as many hours of sleep as when they were younger. Relaxed, deep breathing and herbal teas can be helpful. Warm milk which has the amino acid tryptophan, also a sleep-inducer, can be useful as well.

16. *Fatigue.* The sense of overwhelming fatigue can be hard to beat, but oddly enough one way to counter it is to get more exercise, which both energizes the body and mind and makes it easier to relax when you want to sleep. You can also counter fatigue by participating in activities you really love to do, for which you can muster lots of motivation and energy.

# HORMONE REPLACEMENT THERAPY: THE PROS AND CONS

Over the years, a controversy has been raging on whether or not women in midlife should be taking medication that replaces the hormones that decline at menopause.

Will hormones make you live longer? Will they take ten years off your life? We still don't know, and that's the problem when it comes to figuring out what you want in the long run. Some women feel terrific when they're on *hormone replacement therapy* (HRT); others can't wait to get off the pills. It's for you to decide.

There are many interesting studies that have come out, pro and con, but each woman has to make up her own mind in consultation with her medical doctor. There is not one way for everyone, and you should remember that even if you decide on one course of action, you can always change later on if you find that it's not working for you.

## The History of HRT

Hormone replacement therapy (HRT) was first developed by Dr. Robert Wilson in the late 1960s. At that time, it was known as ERT, or *estrogen replacement therapy.* Dr. Wilson, in his book, *Feminine Forever,* wrote that estrogen was the fountain of youth for midlife women and would restore their vibrant glow and sexuality as nothing else could. Consequently, patients flocked to him in droves, and began his regimen of taking large doses of estrogen.

Within a year, many of these women were diagnosed with endometrial cancer—cancer of the lining of the uterus. Dr. Wilson was censured and his plan denigrated.

But in laboratories and medical research centers all over the country, doctors continued work on the basic precept of Wilson's idea. They thought that they should model their regimen on the natural female cycle, where both estrogen and progesterone work together to enable the lining of the uterus slough off each month. For the first half of the month, they gave estrogen alone, and then, 12 to 14 days into the cycle, they added progesterone. After 25 days, they stopped both hormones, and in a few more days, the patient bled just as though she were having a real period.

Through the years, this administration of HRT has become the gold standard. Women who have had hysterectomies and have no uterus take only estrogen; everyone else takes the combined regimen of estrogen plus *progestin* (synthetic progesterone). Dosages have dropped drastically, and the majority of obstetrician/gynecologists and many family practice doctors recommend HRT to their midlife patients. Not only does it alleviate the signs and signals of menopause, reducing or eliminating hot flashes and vaginal dryness, but it appears to be the most influential factor in preventing osteoporosis because it keeps calcium in the bone and keeps bone mass and density high. It also appears to retain beneficial lipid levels in the blood, and is therefore protective against heart disease.

### Why Is There Reluctance Among Women to Take HRT?

About ten percent of all midlife women in America decide to take HRT, however only twenty percent of those who start the regimen continue. There are a variety of reasons.

1. Many women dislike the idea of having a "period" when they are 50 or 60 years old.

2. If you are taking HRT for your heart and bones, most physicians say you must take it for the rest of your life. Is it wise to medicate a perfectly healthy woman? Are we not leaving ourselves open for possible problems down the line? Since the longest

studies on women taking these hormones last only 14 years or so, it's still too soon to say how safe it is long term.

3. The progestin component of the regimen makes most women feel moody and depressed. This is the hormone responsible for the symptoms of PMS, and some women are terribly sensitive to it.

4. According to several influential studies, progestin seems to increase the risk of breast cancer in certain women. A five-year Swedish study showed that a group taking both estrogen and progesterone had a rate of breast cancer four times as high as those who took no hormones and twice as high as those who took estrogen alone.

   More recent studies have found that natural micronized progesterone, although much more difficult to manufacture and more expensive, seems to create fewer health risks and is tolerated better by patients. The proportion of progesterone used is generally lower in the natural form. However, again, it may be too soon to say what the long-term benefits and risks of this type of therapy are.

5. Estrogen, too, has been associated with increased cancer risk. The most telling factor here is dosage—most of the breast cancers that were seen in hysterectomized women (only taking estrogen) were those whose daily dosage exceeded 1.5 mg. The standard dose is 0.625 mg.; however the medication is manufactured in dosages that go up as high as 2.5 mg.

6. Since the oral administration of HRT has to pass through the gut and the liver, which processes the toxins we take into our bodies, there have been instances of liver tumors and gallbladder disease subsequent to HRT. Both the liver and gallbladder can be affected by estrogen.

7. Hormone replacement therapy can produce a variety of unpleasant side effects, from weight gain and bloating to high blood pressure to headaches.

8. The two hormones also promote fluid retention in the body, which would mean that anyone with conditions exacerbated by excess fluid, such as asthma, migraines, epilepsy, or cardiac or kidney disease would have to be carefully monitored on HRT.

## Dosages and Methods of Taking HRT

You can take HRT in many different forms. Most of the conjugated or natural (animal-based) estrogens are manufactured from pregnant mares' urine. The progesterone can be given in a synthetic or natural form. Let's run these down in order:

1. *Oral, cyclical.* A low dose of a conjugated estrogen (usually .625 Premarin, but there are many other products on the market) is given for the first 25 days of the cycle, and then Provera (a synthetic progestin) is added in doses of 2.5, 5 or 10 mg. for days 12 through 25. You can also take a natural micronized progesterone, a powder compounded into wax-based rectal and vaginal suppositories, oral capsules, or troches which dissolve under the tongue. You take no supplements for days 25 to 28 and then have a "period."

2. *Oral, continuous.* Since one of the benefits of passing through menopause is a cessation of menses, most women are not delighted to learn that they may bleed when they take HRT. So many doctors now prescribe hormones continuously—that is, you take your estrogen daily throughout the month and add the progestin or natural progesterone for the second half of the month. You don't discharge the lining of the uterus this way and the dosages are broken down enough to prevent a precancerous condition from developing. Many women still experience some breakthrough bleeding when they receive a continuos dosage, at least for the first three or four months.

3. *Transdermal patch or gel.* A small, round patch with an estrogen reservoir is attached to the hip or buttock and changed twice weekly. The skin acts as the semipermeable membrane through which the estrogen enters the bloodstream. Progesterone or a progestin must be given separately. This administration bypasses the liver, and seems to be particularly good for the prevention of osteoporosis. However, many doctors feel it doesn't give adequate cardiac protection because it doesn't cause the same lipid changes as the oral variety.

The gel, which dries into a patch, can be applied twice weekly. It is comparable to the transdermal patch in terms of protection.

4. *Estrogen cream.* If your only complaint is vaginal dryness, you can use this topical cream twice a week to enhance lubrication of the vagina and labia. It's important not to apply the cream just before intercourse, since much of it would leak out, obviating its effect.

5. *Subcutaneous implant*. A small estrogen pellet is implanted in the lower abdomen and can be left there for three months to a year (depending on dosage) before it's changed. Progestin or progesterone is also necessary for any woman who has not had a hysterectomy.

## Is HRT for You?

This is not an easy question to answer, and it will depend a great deal on how you feel about the medicalization of an event that is perfectly normal within the context of the aging process. There are good reasons to take HRT and good reasons to avoid it.

You are definitely a good prospect for HRT if:

1. You have had an early surgical menopause. If you have had your uterus and/or ovaries removed in your twenties or thirties, you will have many years of hormonal imbalance before you. This in turn will put you at higher risk for both osteoporosis and heart disease. Hormone replacement is currently considered advisable in this case.

2. You have a strong personal or family history of either osteoporosis or heart disease. If your sisters, your mother, or your grandmother suffered from either of these conditions, you should get as much preventive protection as you can. The results of the Brigham and Women's Hospital ten-year survey of 49,000 nurses show that risk of heart disease can be halved on a regimen of HRT. A more recent study at the University of Pittsburgh showed that in order to glean beneficial effects for your heart, you must take hormones for at least ten years.

3. You are a perfectly healthy peri- or postmenopausal woman, a nonsmoker, within a ten-pound range of your ideal weight who is concerned about her health and is willing to consider medical options to staying well as you age.

You can use HRT with caution if your healthcare provider agrees and will monitor you carefully if:

1. You're a smoker.

2. You are obese (over 20 percent of normal body weight for your height).

3. You suffer from asthma, diabetes, hypertension, migraines, fibrocystic breast disease, or uterine fibroids.

4. You are a DES daughter (your mother took diethylstilbestrol when she was pregnant with you).

You should *not* take HRT if

1. You have any estrogen-dependent cancer such as breast, uterine, or ovarian cancer. (Some physicians extend this to an immediate family history as well.)

2. You have liver or gallbladder disease.

3. You have a history of stroke, deep vein thrombosis or prior pulmonary blockage.

## What Happens If You Change Your Mind About HRT?

The most important consideration in reversing your decision to take HRT is slow withdrawal. If you should find that you are overly worried about this treatment and wish to stop taking it, you should do so with your doctor's guidance to avoid the *rebound effect*, in which your body reacts to the immediate withdrawal of estrogen. The effect is similar to having a surgical menopause: instead of having an entire climacteric of several years to adjust to hormonal imbalances, you experience it within a week or so. This could mean severe hot flashes and vaginal dryness, as well as other menopausal signs. In addition, you could be at increased risk of bone loss and lipid changes. Bone loss after withdrawal in some cases occurs more quickly and more dramatically than it does in women who have never taken HRT at all.

You and your doctor should plan a new schedule to wean you off the medication gradually and, at the same time, you should make certain to keep up with nonmedical treatments (see below) that may help you over the difficult weeks.

## NATURAL WAYS TO STAY HEALTHY DURING MIDLIFE

First, it must be said that there is no substitute for HRT when it comes to protection of your bones and heart. But, having said that, I must add immediately that, by not medicating yourself, you eliminate the anxiety of not knowing what replacement hormones might do to you over many decades. That stress might in and of itself be detrimental to your health.

So what else can you do?

1. *Nutrition*. A well-rounded, low-fat, low-salt, low-sugar, low-meat, low-cholesterol, high complex-carbohydrate, high-fiber diet is the way to go. Eating well will make enormous differences in your lipid levels and will give you the energy to maintain a good exercise program. See Chapter Two for particulars.

- ❏ Add soy products (miso, tempeh and tofu) to your diet. The Japanese suffer very little from the signs and signals of menopause because of the phytoestrogens (estrogens in plants) in their diet.

- ❏ Use brewer's yeast, lecithin, fresh fruit, vegetable juices which are all plant sources of estrogen healthy vitamins and minerals.

- ❏ Eliminate caffeine, alcohol, hot, and spicy foods to reduce or eliminate hot flashes.

- ❏ Insert an egg white or spoonful of nonpasteurized plain yogurt into the vagina to counteract dryness.

- ❏ Drink cranberry or cherry juice for cystitis.

- ❏ Take bee pollen, sold in health food stores as chewable tablets, which is useful for hot flashes.

2. *Exercise*. There is nothing like it! Daily aerobic exercise lowers your risk of cardiovascular disease, builds bone mass, reduces the severity of hot flashes and improves your sexual functioning. Cross training is the best option—you might walk three days a week and swim four days. Or you might alternate jogging with yoga or tai chi chuan. It's a good idea to get a mix of aerobic and non-aerobic activities.

3. *Supplementation*. Make sure you're taking a good multivitamin. In addition, all midlife women should be taking calcium (1000–1500 mg. daily) with half as much magnesium for bone loss.

Other supplements can help with some specific menopausal complaints:

- ❏ B-complex with additional B$_6$, 100 mg. daily (good for hot flashes)

- ❏ Vitamin E (up to 400 IU twice daily) for flashes. Also, as an antioxidant, E has been found to be protective against heart disease. However, if you have diabetes, hypertension or a rheumatic heart condition, you should take no more than 100 mg. daily.

- ❏ Vitamin E oil squeezed from capsule on the vaginal area will help alleviate dryness.

- ❏ Vitamin D to speed absorption of calcium.

- ❏ Evening primrose oil for tender breasts, insomnia, and hot flashes.

- ❏ Vitamin A (10,000 IU twice daily) for excessive menstrual bleeding during perimenopause.

4. *Herbal remedies.* Herbs are the oldest means of healing known to man. In addition, they provide nutrients we often miss in our over-processed foods. The following is a small list of herbs you might consider taking at midlife.

- ❏ *Ginseng* and *dong quai* (Cimicifuga racemosa) both useful for hot flashes.

- ❏ *Yellow melilot* (as a tea) for insomnia.

- ❏ *Horsetail,* or *dong quai* tea for excessive bleeding during perimenopause.

- ❏ *Chaste tree* and *monk's pepper* (Vitex agnus castus) and *salvia leaves* as tea for hot flashes.

- ❏ Teas made of *fenugreek, black cohosh, sarsaparilla,* or *gota kola* for hot flashes.

5. *Homeopathic remedies.* Homeopathy is a system of medicine based on the idea that "like can cure like." That is, two types of similar discomforts cannot exist in the body at the same time. A small amount of a toxic substance can stimulate the body's natural attempt to restore balance. Given the right remedy, the body cures itself. You may want to start your pursuit of this medicine by having a consultation with a homeopathic physician, who will be able to give you specific remedies suitable to your discomforts, as well as to your body type and emotional make-up. Homeopathic remedies are available in most health-food stores, so that you can read the lists of symptoms and match them to your own.

There are over 100 remedies for hot flashes alone, and 20 for flashes with perspiration, but the three most common used for relief of menopausal signs are *sepia, lachesis,* and *natrum mur.*

6. *Over-the-counter vaginal lubricants.* You can purchase a variety of lubricants at your local drugstore to counteract vaginal dryness, including Replens, Astroglide, Gyne-Moistrin or Calendula cream. *Never* use an oil-based lubricant such as baby oil, solid shortening, or vaseline with rubber contraceptives because these can damage and destroy latex condoms.

7. *Mind power.* A variety of techniques, from visualization to meditation to self-hypnosis can be excellent for changing the way that menopausal ailments affect you. If you change your mind, you can often change your body.

8. *Pursue an activity that will fulfill mind and body.* Yoga and tai chi chuan are two ancient healthful practices that discipline you and calm you at the same time. By practicing a choreographed set of postures or "forms," you achieve the quiet awareness of being calm within yourself. These two meditative arts train the body to be resilient, enduring and flexible as they train the mind to clear out the cobwebs of stress—and both are reputed to increase longevity.

# WHAT YOU NEED TO KNOW ABOUT
# HYSTERECTOMY AND OOPHORECTOMY

Hysterectomy is the surgical removal of the uterus, and usually the cervix as well. Oophorectomy is the removal of your ovaries, either alone or with the uterus, fallopian tubes, and cervix. After an oophorectomy, you cannot bear children because you no longer produce eggs. You also go through an immediate surgical menopause, losing your hormonal source of estrogen overnight.

As many as one-third of American women have a hysterectomy before they turn 60, and forty to fifty percent of them have their ovaries removed at the same time. This is the most frequently performed operation in America—approximately 600,000 of these procedures take place every year, and that's not even counting the outpatient procedures that go unreported. In Germany, the hysterectomy rate is 11 percent; in England, it's 14 percent. Why are doctors in our country so dedicated to performing this operation?

The male medical establishment has long misunderstood the nature—both psychological and spiritual—of a woman's reproductive organs. They aren't just meant for having babies! Keeping all your organs, if they are basically healthy, is helpful to living longer. Removal of a woman's ovaries is a form of castration, and can result in disastrous health complications such as osteoporosis, heart disease, and complete loss of libido. Removal of the uterus may cause surrounding organs to shift as they fill in the space left by the excised uterus. The bladder, rectum, or vagina may become displaced and complicated surgery may be required to restore them. In addition, hysterectomy can wreak havoc with your self-image. This is not simply another piece of your body like your toe or your ear; for many women it is the symbol of their femininity.

## Diagnosis Is Essential to Determine Whether or Not You Need Surgery

The rates of hysterectomy are decreasing slowly due to advances in diagnostic medicine. Today, a woman who is bleeding uncontrollably or whose Pap test shows an abnormality or who has a mass that can be felt during a medical exam is not immediately sent for surgery.

Rather, she would first have a *hysteroscopic examination* or an *endometrial biopsy*, so that the tissue of the uterine cavity could be examined.

She might have a *dilation and curettage* (D&C), where the lining of the uterus is scraped off and then examined in the laboratory for abnormal thickening, cancer, or polyps.

She might have a *cervical biopsy* or *colposcopy* to examine her cervix.

And with *carbon dioxide laparoscopy*, a surgeon can examine the whole interior of the pelvic cavity through an opening no bigger than a dime and determine just what's wrong.

It used to be a foregone conclusion that you should have a hysterectomy if you had uterine fibroids that caused pain, bleeding, or repeated miscarriage or infertility; or if you had endometriosis. Today, most physicians will use stop-gap methods for fibroids which naturally shrink at menopause anyway (fibroids grow under the influence of estrogen), and laser surgery and hormonal therapies are the most common treatments for endometriosis.

## Good Reasons for Having Hysterectomy or Oophorectomy

The decision as to whether to hysterectomize or oophorectomize a woman, therefore, should be made only as a last resort, if it will in fact save her life or relieve disabling symptoms. Surgery is absolutely necessary to prevent an established cancer from spreading, or because no other method has been able to control severe bleeding. Another good reason for a hysterectomy is a prolapsed uterus, where the pelvic floor has so weakened that the organ has fallen down and protrudes through the cervix and sometimes the vagina.

The operation is usually performed through an abdominal incision, although if the reason for the surgery is prolapse, it can be done vaginally, and this approach offers a quicker recovery.

## Recuperating from Surgery

For most women, it will take six weeks just to get back on your feet again. During this time you should do no heavy lifting or hard work. You can start doing some gentle exercises to get your abdominal muscles back in tone after this time, but you should progress very slowly. You may feel that urinating and defecating feel different because of the altered placement of your organs.

You may also have many mixed feelings about resuming your sex life. Physically, it's important to make sure your surgeon shortens your vagina as little as possible so that you can accommodate your partner's penis comfortably. You will certainly need to use a vaginal lubricant if you have chosen not to take HRT, and this aid may enhance sexual pleasure whether you're on hormones or not.

How you feel about your femininity and sexuality at this point will very much depend on your attitudes before the surgery. There is nothing different about you as a sexual person now other than the fact that you lack a uterus. You are still as sexy and desirable; just remember that it may take a few months before intercourse feels good again. It's wonderful to be able to experiment with nonpenetrative sex—and this is a good excuse to try oral and manual techniques with your partner.

If you have had your ovaries removed and you feel no desire for sex whatsoever, you can speak to your physician about testosterone replacement. This male hormone, which women also produce (although in much smaller amounts than men), is what gives you your sex drive. Supplementing it could make a big difference in the way you feel about making love after surgery.

## HOW GOOD CAN YOU FEEL AT MIDLIFE?

This journey to the second half of your life is certainly not only about hormones. It is, rather, a personal passage that involves much psychological, emotional, and spiritual change. A woman of 50 or so can be like a runner hitting her stride. No longer jogging in time with anyone else, she can sprint away and take the field. But she has to have the drive, the guts, and the motivation to break out of the pack and go it on her own.

At 50, you may be freer of family obligations than you were at 30 or 40. You may be more financially secure and have fewer distractions. You can do what you like, when you like. The main challenge is to believe in the beneficial possibilities of change.

## Restructuring Old Patterns Can Be Good for You

Menopause occurs at such a seminal time in a woman's life. Your children are nearly grown or already out of the house, or perhaps, in this tight economy, moving back into the house with children of their own. Empty nest syndrome becomes refilled nest syndrome. Because women in America typically outlive their spouses by six and a half years, and often marry men who are older than themselves, you may be widowed, suddenly robbed of your lifelong companion, and on your own again. Or you may be going through a divorce, as many couples discover at this time that it was the children who kept them together. Or you may find yourself alone because the man in your life is going through a personal crisis and says he needs his freedom. You may have elderly parents to care for; you may have close friends who move away or become ill and die, reminding you of your own mortality.

Left to your own devices or newly crowned head-of-the-household Role, you are the person in charge. What do you do with this power?

This is a time to reassess all your roles. Are you still a caregiver, a nurturer with no one to take care of? You can mentor younger people at work, pointing them in the right direction. Do you feel as though you haven't reached your creative potential? You can go back to school, travel, quit a dull job or start a business of your own.

There are women who find all these choices overwhelming. The comfortable patterns of life have suddenly shattered. It's easy to feel uncertain as to what if anything can be salvaged. And there are women who become so depressed, it can be difficult for them to think about new ways to enjoy the aging process. But it doesn't have to be that way.

## Learning What Your True Potential Can Be

Let me tell you about Laura, one of my patients. She's a school-teacher in her mid-fifties, a vibrant, interesting woman. As she started her passage through menopause, her 20-year marriage split up, her youngest child left for college, and she suddenly found herself having panic attacks. She was worried that time had passed her by and wanted desperately to change her situation. When she came to me, we talked about the stress in her life and how she might think about reducing it. "I'm not a person who can sit and contemplate my navel," she protested when I suggested meditation.

"What do you love to do?" I asked. "What could you do that would take your mind off everything else?" "I'm crazy about dancing," she confided. "But I don't have a partner." I suggested that she shouldn't let that stop her.

Laura found a local dance club that met twice a week and started line dancing. She got really good at it, and aside from the physical exercise making her feel better, her social life expanded. She stopped drinking caffeine, which helped her hot flashes, and had a glass of wine only once a week. She increased her intake of vitamins and although she opted not to take HRT, she started reading up on herbs and homeopathic therapy. Her mood swings and anxiety tapered off, and as she started sleeping better at night, she regained a lot of her old self-confidence. When school was out, she took a trip by herself to Greece and Turkey, two countries she'd always wanted to visit. When I last saw her, she told me she loved her life, and was delighted to have about fifty more years of it ahead of her to look forward to.

## The Next Fifty Years

Goal planning is essential if you're going to discover what you really can do with your life—for yourself and others. Remember that giving yourself at least ten more years of life means that you have to fill them meaningfully. As you understand that you deserve to please yourself as well as others, you can choose some self-fulfilling as well as altruistic pursuits. Here are a few suggestions:

1. *Give up the submissive role.* For the first time in your life, you are the captain of your fate. You're mature enough to be a peer along with your partner, whether it's the beginning of a new relationship or a long-lasting one. You have a stronger say in the decisions affecting your destiny than at any other time in your life.

2. *Redefine your role in life.* Here is an opportunity for you to redefine your role in life, into one that has the drama, creativity, accomplishments, independence about which you've only dreamt till now. Never before in your life has it been so true that you have no one to answer to but yourself. "Freedom," as the Kris Kristoferson song says, "is just another word for nothin' left to lose." Menopause is not an end; it's a glorious beginning, if you choose to make it so.

3. *Enjoy a new sense of adventure.* You're freer than ever to change your career, to join new groups of individuals whose interests you've always wanted to explore, to travel to exotic places for your vacation, to be more candid and honest than you've ever been before. Finally, the world is yours to explore, to enjoy, to learn from, to gain recognition from, as never before.

4. *Enjoy sex as never before.* You can now become more independent in your relationship, or enjoy the sense of independence of living alone, without being accountable to anyone but yourself. Married or single, you can take more responsibility for having your sexual needs satisfied. No need to play the role of the submissive female—you can confidently communicate how and where you want to be touched and stroked. Taking initiative in the bedroom, when done with mature sensitivity, can be more fun for you *and* your partner.

5. *Share the responsibilities of care taking.* If you have to take care of ailing parents, put this in perspective and don't let this sense of responsibility overshadow your life. You're more skilled as a caretaker now, more effective at managing your time. Look for other resources with whom to share this unavoidable responsibility: siblings or other relatives, close friends of your parents, community and government agencies. Don't let old patterns of guilt resurface. Rather than the lone savior of your increasingly helpless parents, see yourself as a confident and effective manager of resources. Share the wealth of responsibilities. And continue to enjoy the rest of your life!

# ANTIAGING
## SEXUALITY AND
## REPRODUCTIVE HEALTH

## CHAPTER 6

As long as you're alive, you are a sexual person, no matter what your age. You have drives and passions, and needs to touch and be touched. Women, more than men, seem to tune into their sexuality more as they mature, and the more sexual they allow themselves to feel, the younger they can feel. The more that we as a society can downplay the idea of sex being merely for the young, the more we can reclaim our rights to love, to live, and to pass on a warm and intimate legacy to the next generation.

In this chapter, we'll explore longevity as it relates to sex, and also to your reproductive health. Your uterus, vagina, ovaries, and breasts are distinctly important, not just in terms of your femininity, but also as they relate to your general health. So whether you want to have a baby at 40 or become a sexual guru at 60, you need to take very good care of your sexual organs and your sexual spirit as well.

## YOUR SEXUALITY AS YOU AGE

When we begin our sexual lives, as children or young adults, we are fumbling and confused—about our bodies, about the various feelings we have, and about what sexuality is in reality.

As we mature, we have the luxury of approaching our sexuality in a much more holistic fashion. No longer need we be concerned with being a perfect "10" or performing brilliantly all night long. We can, if we're open enough to accept new ideas, think of sex as a way to know ourselves and one another better.

## How to Keep Sex Alive over the Years

If you are a mature adult and have been in a long-term relationship for several decades, you know that it isn't always easy to feel the same spontaneity or excitement that you felt when you first met your mate. Living with a partner means that you have to accommodate another person's needs, whims, and desires, and at the same time, that you have to find a way to get what you want for yourself. It can be difficult to achieve a balance between two sets of sexual feelings, but it's worth doing. If you think of it as play rather than work (because, after all, sex *is* adult play), you'll succeed most of the time.

If you're not currently partnered, you have a different challenge. Single women in our society tread a fine line between being valued only for their sexuality and being regarded as asexual after they pass a certain age. There's no reason for this other than prejudice and myth. The key is that you must take charge of your sexuality and let others know how you expect to be treated. A woman of twenty may find that it's important for her growth as a person to be celibate; a woman of 60 may find that she has at last comprehended the true meaning of intimacy, orgasm, masturbation, and ecstasy.

The nice thing about sexuality is that it's always changing, and you can change with it.

## The Magic of Communication

If you don't talk about sex, it becomes an act, just the joining of two bodies without thought or consideration. If you ignore the various anxieties and problems that may have stymied your sexual life, you end up avoiding intimacy and eroding your relationship.

Think first about what drew you to your partner when you met. At that time, before you ever touched, you had to communicate with words. You had to introduce yourself, open yourself up to your partner's values and ideas, and entertain the notion of accepting someone else's philosophy and way of living. This was interesting! This started your juices flowing. As you became involved with the other person and your physical attraction grew, you felt an overwhelming desire to get closer. But you approached each other cautiously, step by step, so as not to spoil something that was new and growing.

That's the way to think about communicating even if you've been together for twenty or thirty years. People are always changing: hopefully, if you are able to appreciate the direction you've both taken in life, you'll be able to be attracted to your partner all over again.

A successful sexual relationship thrives on trust that is built over the years. It comes from a willingness to be vulnerable and open to explore one another's fears, hopes, and dreams. You have to earn each other's trust—and that means being careful about protecting your partner and what you know about him. It's all too easy, when you're angry or frustrated with him, to start a verbal warfare based on his vulnerabilities.

In talking about the way you feel, you can encourage him to talk more as well. You can also encourage him to pay more attention to your sexual likes and dislikes if you actually come right out and let him know what they are. In most relationships, unfortunately, sexual development takes place much more quickly than emotional disclosure. Men and women bare their bodies more quickly than they bare their souls. And in those relationships that last, sexual patterns develop that are difficult to alter. Once these patterns are set, it becomes harder to discuss changes, because we sense both our own and our partner's vulnerabilities so keenly.

If you want to change something that's happening between you in the bedroom, select a time to talk when sex isn't the issue, maybe during a long ride in the car or when you're taking a coffee break between some Saturday chores. Be aware that your partner won't take criticism of his style or technique well when he's in the midst of a passionate encounter. You want to be gentle with his feelings just as you would like him to be with yours.

How can you break through the silence barrier and really communicate better to enjoy more mature sex?

1. *Learn to accommodate and negotiate your different sex drives.* There is no question that people at the beginning of a relationship tend to think about sex more and act on their thoughts than those who've

been together for years. And as time passes, it becomes clear that one partner tends to have a drive toward more frequent sex and the other's interest is more on the back burner. In dysfunctional couples, one pursues and the other keeps the pursuer at a distance. The longer this goes on, the more likelihood that problems will occur as one partner becomes more needy and risks feeling rejected.

To communicate better, give each other breathing space. You have to accept that you aren't going to be in accord all the time, but every once in a while, you can allow your partner his preference. If you keep an open mind about sex, you may find that you can enjoy your differences. Sometimes one of you will play the leader, and the other, the follower. Then you reverse. It can be a lot of fun looking at sex the way your partner sees it as long as you don't have to accommodate to his style all the time.

2. *Learn to negotiate.* It can be very stressful if one of you wants to hang from the chandelier and the other is content with the missionary position. We all have fantasies and personal sexual styles, but in a relationship, it's important to acknowledge the other person's style. This is not to say that you should bend to it all the time. Good sexual negotiation means a balance—whether it's about time, place, or who initiates the activities.

3. *Discuss what you like and don't like.* If you've never said how much you like it when he bites the inside of your thigh, go ahead and say it. It's wonderful to get feedback and compliments, and he may respond in kind if you're more verbal about what you like in bed. (Or he may not, because men tend to feel embarrassed about expressing themselves sexually—just don't push him and see what may transpire if you're patient.)

If you really don't like something that occurs between you sexually, whether it bores you or hurts you, find a time to convey that. Without being punitive or demanding, you can make your wishes known. If you phrase this as, "I'd rather do this. . ." or "could you tone that down a little?" it won't come out too harshly.

4. *Use "hand" language.* You don't have to talk all the time. You can simply guide your partner's hands and mouth to where you'd like them. A little guidance in the right direction can be helpful without being critical.

5. *Be honest.* There's no sense in lying about sex, because what you feel will come out nonverbally even if you don't say it in words. If you value your partner, you will come clean, even if it's hard to speak. Clearly there are times when you shouldn't say anything—you might not want to share a homosexual fantasy or information about an affair you once had because of hurting his feelings. But the truth does matter when it pertains to things that really matter between you.

## Overcoming Myths About Sex as We Age

If you've been clinging to old myths about sex that are keeping you from really enjoying yourself and your partner, it's time you got rid of them.

*Myth* 1: Great sex should be spontaneous.

*Truth*: It's nice when you come together like two stars colliding, but in the real world, that doesn't happen very often. Planning sex and making dates with your partner allows for the anticipating and whetting of your appetite. It also allows you to take care of practical issues like childcare, housecare, work deadlines, and your own fatigue and exhaustion after a hard day.

*Myth* 2: Great sex equals a great relationship.

*Truth*: There are many couples who have totally dysfunctional relationships and can only communicate physically. There are also loving couples who have sexual problems. Commitment, love, and mutual respect are much more important than how many orgasms you give each other.

*Myth* 3: Simultaneous orgasm is the best kind.

*Truth*: It can really be more mutually pleasurable for one of you to come first, and then the other. This way, you get to enjoy your own moment in the sun and then concentrate on your partner's. It's also a relief not to be thinking about a goal that may be impossible to reach.

*Myth* 4: If you're married, you shouldn't masturbate.

*Truth*: Masturbation is a personal activity that allows you to give yourself pleasure. It is not inimical to partnered sex—as a matter of fact, you can show your partner better what you like in bed after figuring it out by yourself.

*Myth* 5: If you're pregnant or have just had a child, you can forget about sex.

*Truth*: It was sex that got you there in the first place! This is a time to really develop your sexuality with that of your partner. If he's afraid of hurting your baby, show him some pictures of the female anatomy and explain that the fetus is cushioned and protected by your body. If the two of you feel uncomfortable with each other because you are locked in the belief that mothers have to be motherly (and therefore not sexual), begin by touching and caressing in a nonsexual, nonthreatening way. This may lead you to an understanding of how right and good being physical together can be, both during pregnancy and afterward.

If you or your partner is having problems because of your changed body image, take a good look at yourself naked in the mirror. The beauty of the female form is only enhanced during pregnancy. It's just a question of getting used to yourself in a different form. The function is just the same!

*Myth* 6: If you don't have multiple orgasms, you aren't very sexy.

*Truth*: Some completely inorgasmic women have wonderfully satisfying sex lives. It all depends on what you enjoy. Cuddling, hugging, and kissing can produce a wave of delight as intense as a clitoral orgasm for certain women. As it happens, most people who do become multiply orgasmic achieve this when they're older and have more experience in exploring their sexuality.

*Myth* 7: If you trust your partner, you'll share all your fantasies and act them out.

*Truth*: All of us have great imaginations, but this doesn't mean we have to act on them. It can be harmful and disappointing to try to accomplish in real life all the various things that turn us on mentally. Your partner may or may not want to share the inner workings of your mind; you must use careful judgment before divulging some of your wilder fantasies.

*Myth* 8: If you fake orgasm, it will make your partner happy.

*Truth*: If you aren't having orgasms and want to, you should discuss this with your partner. There's no point in pretending that you've reached a climax just to please your partner, or to end a less than satisfactory sexual encounter. It's possible that you'll respond better to oral or manual stimulation or that you might come more easily if you experimented with a vibrator or other sex toy. If you stop faking and start paying attention to your own body, you may find that you respond in a much more relaxed fashion—and actually have an orgasm!

*Myth* 9: If your partner is having problems with his erections, he's not attracted to you any more.

*Truth*: All men have sexual anxieties at one time or another, and sometimes, they're just plain tired and their body doesn't respond as they'd like it to. A penis isn't a piece of plumbing, it's an integral part of a man. You don't need a hard penis for lovemaking, which is something else that's nice to realize as you get older. Men can have orgasms without erections, and it's not necessary for them to ejaculate each time. The two of you can also do all sorts of things that don't involve penetration—sucking, kissing, licking, nibbling—and still have a wonderful time.

## The Seasons of a Woman's Life

In your thirties and forties, after your family is pretty well established, you can start thinking about sexuality as separate from reproduction. This in turn can open up a new world of sensuality and feeling. As you pass menopause, and don't need to be concerned with contraception or a monthly period, the whole event can be much more focussed on pure pleasure.

Many women shift into high gear sexually when they reach their fiftieth birthday. As estrogens decline in the body (see Chapter 5), they feel more responsive to the androgens which arouse the libido. For other women, who may not have enjoyed their sex lives in earlier decades, sexuality can be a challenge, although satisfaction doesn't necessarily decrease at this time.

At this time of life, a vaginal lubricant is often a necessity, to mimic the natural lubricants women no longer produce in abundance. There are great products available in your local drugstore without prescription, that may restore the zing to your sex life.

As we all age, it takes longer for both men and women to become aroused. A man in his seventies may require 30 to 40 minutes of foreplay to become fully erect. But this is really beneficial for both partners since foreplay becomes anytime play, and is just as stimulating as the penetrative act.

According to a survey of 800 elderly couples, 75 percent of women in their 80s say that their love-making has actually improved over time. So as you look forward to ten extra years of healthy life, you can anticipate your sexuality growing and expanding as well.

## Why Sex Improves with Age

We have deeper sexual needs as we get older. Someone described it once as the difference between the rush of downhill skiing and the pleasure of cross-country skiing, where you get to pause and watch the scenery go by. When we reach our forties and fifties, it's not necessary to race to the finish. Instead, we can enjoy one another fully—our bodies, personalities, senses of humor, or senses of failure—and explore in depth what it means to be creative, nurturing, empowering, and sexual in bed or out of it. All these facets of us converge, as we age, in a more holistic and spiritual type of bonding. After all, there is no other event in life that makes two bodies into one. And as we become one with a partner, we learn that we are perhaps part of something larger—the cosmos or universe—in this act of give and take, of learning and growth.

Each decade of life can bring greater sexual satisfaction. As we let go of preoccupation with perfomance and become more sensual instead of just sexual, we can finally relax. Women can become more confident about their ability to initiate sex as they see their partners become less anxious to lie back and be taken care of. This affords greater opportunity for creative play and longer lasting sexual encounters.

In a landmark study of 80- to 102-year-old individuals in a nursing home conducted by Bernard Starr and Marcella Weiner in 1981, it was found that the most elderly individuals felt that sex was an integral part of their lives. They felt that it enhanced their physical and emotional health, and that it could improve with age. It gave them a reason to get up in the morning, to look well and feel well. The men and women who were most interested in intimacy and sexual activity said that they had always liked sex—and prior enjoyment seems to be a big key to retaining pleasure as we age.

Our sexuality is like a muscle: If you don't use it, you lose it.

## What You Can Do to Enhance Your Sexuality

Exercise is terrific for sex, and sex is terrific exercise. Research shows that women who engage in some form of exercise three to ten hours a week are more easily aroused, have more orgasms, and are more confident about their sexuality. Here are some easy exercises that will keep you sexually fit.

1. *Kegel Exercises.* You might have been taught these after childbirth, but they're terrific for you at any age. They will help prevent incontinence in later life as well. In order to do a Kegel, pretend that you are sitting on a toilet, releasing the flow of urine. Then, think about stopping the flow by contracting the muscles in the vaginal area. You'll also feel your anal sphincter tighten up. Do a set of ten of these three times a day and they will give you and your partner a great deal of pleasure.

2. *Arm flexes.* To increase flexibility in your arms, to hold yourself up in bed, or to take the weight of a partner, here's what to do. Straighten your arms in front of you, grab your left wrist with your right hand and extend your arms over your head. Pull them slightly backward until you feel a pull under your armpits. Hold for a count of five, then relax. Repeat five times.

3. *Abdominal curls.* To strengthen abdominal muscles, which will give a firm tone to the pelvic area, do the following: Lie on your back with knees bent and hands linked behind your neck. Slowly bring your head and shoulders up until they are about four inches off the floor. Hold for a count of three, relax and repeat several times. Start with ten of these if you aren't in shape and work your way up to thirty slowly.

4. *Hip and groin stretch.* Sit on the floor with the soles of your feet touching, knees out to either side. Reach for your ankles as you press your elbows against the insides of your knees. Now bend forward

slightly and gently push your knees toward the floor. Don't bounce, but hold in the posture for a count of ten. Relax, and repeat ten times. Be gentle and don't stretch beyond your limits.

Another good groin stretch starts with your legs crossed tailor style in front of you. Reach your arms out as you lean forward until you feel a pull in your hips. Relax and repeat five times more.

Experimentation is another way to enhance your sex life. If you always do it in the same place and in the same way, change your mind in order to change your situation. There's no reason to stop fooling around in the back seat just because you've passed your fiftieth birthday. Your sexuality can help you feel younger as you gain the willingness to try new things.

Ecstasy is what we're all looking for, and rarely find. If you have no expectation of delirious delights and you stumble into a  wonderful, tumultuous situation with your partner, so much the better. Sex is sometimes quiet and reflective, sometimes funny and casual. But whatever it is, it's yours. And will be for the rest of your life. Enjoy what comes and you will find yourself looking ten years younger and maybe even extending your lifespan in the bargain.

## YOUR BREASTS AND HOW TO CARE FOR THEM

The female breast is an amazing organ—part sexual, part giver of nourishment. It is one of the first indications that a young girl is becoming a woman, and may be cause for simultaneous pride and embarrassment. A woman may flaunt her breasts in a courtship ritual, cover them up when she's feeling insecure, enjoy them with a partner during the sexual act, and bond with her baby as she senses the reflex which allows her milk to flow. In later life, her breasts may change shape and contour, but they still retain their allure and importance as a symbol of femininity.

### How Is the Breast Structured?

The breast can be understood as being like a sponge with large interconnecting pockets containing milk glands and fat globules. It is interspersed throughout with blood vessels and covered with skin. Interwoven, semi-elastic fibrous ligaments hold the architecture of the breast together. The milk glands are a cluster of tiny grape-like cells whose function is to produce breast milk, which comes down to the nipple via a series of ducts. The only muscles in the breast are the erectile tissue in the nipples, but the breasts themselves sit on the surface of the pectoral muscles of the chest.

The breast may change size and shape radically during pregnancy and lactation due to the increase in pituitary hormones. The skin stretches tightly over the fat and milk ducts, giving the breasts a lift. Many small-breasted women say that they never were as happy as when they were feeding their babies—not just because of the intimate nursing experience but also because of the cosmetic enhancement of their breasts. And large-breasted women, who often complain about having so much tissue because of the difficulties it can pose while sleeping, jogging or exercising, often claim that when they were breastfeeding, they felt truly appreciated for their generous endowment.

When you no longer lactate, the breast changes again. It may revert to its former size and shape, or it may get slightly smaller. Many women find that by the time they reach their forties, the skin is no longer as elastic, nor does the breast sit up as high on the pectoral ledge. At menopause, because of the rapid decline in estrogen, there is less collagen to keep the structure of the breast intact, so it falls a bit. As the ratio of lean muscle tissue to fat changes, the breast tends to become softer. Benign cysts and irregular densities in the breast tissue may become more prominent at this time.

The breast, like every other organ, needs good preventive care. Here are three simple suggestions for healthy breasts:

1. Reduce the fat in your diet.

2. Enjoy daily exercise, which will increase circulation in the breasts as well as throughout your body.

3. Supplement your nutrition with additional vitamin A or beta carotene, $B_6$, and E with selenium.

## Why Are You More Susceptible to Breast Cancer After Menopause?

We're not completely sure why women become more susceptible to breast cancer after menopause, but one probable reason is the time factor. The more years you have to absorb carcinogens in your food and environment, the more likely your body is to store it and let it do its work on various tissues. The chemicals we're exposed to are secreted through our bodily fluids—sweat, saliva, breast secretions, and cervical fluid among others. Over time, as these chemicals travel through the breast tissue, they may affect surrounding cells and cause abnormal growth.

Then, too, some cancers are estrogen-dependent, so the more years you've produced estrogen in your body, the more likely it is that a surfeit of this hormone may adversely affect your organs.

## Learn the Difference Between Benign Lumps and Cancer

Most breast abnormalities and cancers originate in the milk ducts, but not every unusual growth is dangerous. Toward the end of any normal menstrual cycle, most women have kernel-sized breast granules that can be felt on self-examination. Fibrocystic breast disease is not a life-threatening condition, nor is cystic mastitis, where many different-sized tender cysts appear in the breast. Some may actually grow to the size of peanuts. They may be tender and cause breast soreness, but they are quite normal and related to the ovulation process.

Approximately 60 to 80 percent of all breast lumps removed are harmless; thankfully, in these days of sophisticated breast aspiration and biopsy, and stereotactic mammograms which are minimally invasive, much less unnecessary radical surgery is being done.

Cancerous growths are usually hard and painless and are unaffected by your monthly cycle. Benign lumps, on the other hand, are soft, tender and filled with fluid, and may be particularly tender and painful just before your period.

However, you should make no decision on your own. If you feel anything that is not normal for your breast, call your gynecologist at once and have him or her check it out.

## Breast Cancer Risk—What You Need to Know

Although genetic predisposition is a big factor, 85 percent of women diagnosed with breast cancer have no family history of the disease. Only if the cancer occurred in several close relatives at a young age and in both breasts is it likely to be genetic. Food additives, pesticides, pollution, and high-fat diets are actually the chief culprits. Because American women have a typically high-fat diet (most consume about 37 to 40 percent of their daily calories in fat), they are more at risk than, say, Japanese women, who eat a low-fat diet. Eating as they do, American women are in jeopardy because carcinogenic chemicals are easily stored in fat tissue.

Let's look at the high-risk factors you can avoid:

1. Smoking.
2. Consuming over 2 oz. of alcohol daily.
3. Consuming over 30 percent of your calories from fat.
4. Absence of antioxidant vitamins A, C, and E in your diet.
5. Absense of fiber in your diet.
6. Family history of breast cancer.

And some you can't avoid:

7. First menstrual period before your eleventh birthday (meaning that you've been exposed to estrogens for a longer span of time).
8. Childlessness, or first child after you were 30 (again, meaning more exposure to estrogen without "breaks" for pregnancies and nursing).
9. Over age 50.
10. Menopause after age 50.

Five of these risk factors are preventable; all you have to do is make a few lifestyle changes. The first is diet—review Chapter Two if you have any questions about what to eat. The second is smoking and drinking, these are two destructive habits that affect so many of your body's tissues and will absolutely reduce your longevity. The third is preventive examinations—both your own monthly self-exam, your yearly physician's exam, and your mammogram.

## BSE (Breast Self-Exam)

Breast self-examination is a fast, easy, cost-free method of keeping yourself healthy. It's a great habit to get into and puts you a step ahead in your decision to live ten years longer. So many women have discovered a pea-sized tumor at home, which means that they are catching the cancer early, before it has had a chance to spread.

It takes roughly from two to eight years for what begins as a microcosmic lump to become large enough to feel. Although you may be visiting your gynecologist once a year, the lump may not be palpable until a few months after your visit or after your last mammogram. So when you take charge of your own health, you take charge of your life as well.

WHEN IS THE BEST TIME FOR BSE? The best time is a couple of days after your period, if you're still menstruating, or, if you're past menopause, on a convenient day when you'll remember, such as the first of the month. Prior to your period, the hormonal stimulation that enlarges the milk glands may interfere with an accurate reading of your BSE.

WHY DO WOMEN AVOID BSE? Some women, particularly those at high risk, are terrified that they will feel something, and therefore avoid that ten minutes once a month that they could invest in better preventive health. They may take the head-in-the-sand approach, thinking, "If it's there, I don't want to know about it." Others are of the "It won't happen to me" school, and still others think that the procedure is too complicated and they don't know what they're feeling for anyway.

The point is, you don't have to make your own diagnosis. All you have to do is become familiar with your body. If you know what it feels like when it's well, it will be easy for you to understand when something is different. So let me explain it easily and simply.

HOW TO DO YOUR BSE. Before starting on your breasts, practice on the back of your hand. Rotate two fingers around one spot, becoming familiar with the bones and tendons under the skin. Then, using the same procedure, become familiar with the feel of your breasts. That way, if some irregularity persists over a month or so, you'll know that it needs medical attention. Ninety percent of the lumps you'll feel are probably noncancerous and will most likely be more apparent during the late part of your cycle and will probably disappear when your menstrual flow is complete. Those that persist beyond are the ones that need medical attention.

Imagine that your breast is the face of a clock with the nipple as the center. Starting at high noon, using the flat surfaces of your fingers, feel down from the outer limit of the breast (under the collar bone, under the arm, under the curve of the breast, across from the breastbone) into the nipple at each hour. You don't want to glide over the surface: Make sure your fingers press down so that the skin moves with the fingers. If there is an irregularity in your breast, you can feel it between your fingers as well as under them.

Larger-breasted women can use two hands, with one supporting the breast and the other doing the palpation. Then reverse to do the other side of the breast. Smaller-breasted women can use the opposite-side hand to examine the breast while the other arm is raised, resting on the back of the neck.

Make sure you also use overlapping circles so that you cover not just the breast tissue but everything around it as well. Your breast should feel slightly different when you get to the milk ducts at the areola around your nipple—there will be a more granular texture to them and they should move easily beneath your fingers.

You should perform your exam first in the shower, when your breasts are soapy and slippery. When you come out, stand in front of the mirror and look at both breasts and nipples to be sure there is no change in them. Most women normally have uneven sized and shaped breasts—you just want to make sure that they retain those particular sizes and shapes from month to month. There should be no fissures or clefts in the nipple, no discharge coming out of the nipple, and the size of both areolas should be comparable.

Next, raise both arms over your head and look at the breasts again, head on and side to side, for changes in shape. Finally, lean forward from your waist with your arms straight out so that your breasts hang free. In this position, you'll be able to notice dimples or distortions in the breast tissue.

Now lie down with a pillow under the shoulder of the breast you're examining and do the exam again with the breast dry.

How Do You Know What to Feel for? The first few times you examine yourself, you're likely to discover a few irregularities that have probably been there for years. You might notice bony joints or cartilage junctions, extra breast tissue, fatty growths, or sebaceous cysts. These are all normal. If you've recently lost a lot of weight or if you have large, pendulous breasts, you're apt to find two areas of thicker, fibrous tissue in both breasts. Each side will feel like there is a band of rope where the bottom of your breast attaches to the chest wall. You may also feel a thickening at the upper outer quadrant of your breasts, and as long as it's equal on both sides, it's normal. However, if you feel it only on one side, give your physician a call and have it checked out.

Why might you suspect that anything is wrong, either during your examination or any other time you look at your breast? You should see your doctor at once if:

❒ You have discharge from your nipple.

❒ You notice a change in the color or texture of the breast or nipple area.

❒ Your nipple becomes inverted.

❒ You notice a fixed lump or thickening either in the breast or under your arm.

### Mammograms: The Best Breast Cancer Prevention as You Age

Since 1990, government funding of breast cancer research has soared from $87 million to over $410 million. Women's political action groups have helped to make the media respond to this significant statistic: One in nine women will contract breast cancer during her lifetime.

Preventive care is the first and best treatment. This means some attention to your diet and exercise regimes, monthly breast self-exams from puberty throughout life; and a yearly checkup to have your physician perform this exam. A yearly mammogram is essential after age 50; prior to that, the American Cancer Society recommends that you have a baseline mammogram at 39, and then biannually until you're 50, or annually if you have a family history of the disease or if you've had a hysterectomy and are on estrogen replacement.

Recently, the National Cancer Institute has disputed the frequent use of mammograms under the age of 50, saying they aren't cost-effective. But what this actually means is that insurers don't want to pay for most wellness care, and the number of breast cancers detected before menopause is much lower than after menopause.

But this is not a reason to discontinue such important care. Remember that each year, there are 180,000 new cases of breast cancer and 46,000 deaths—and some of these do occur in women under the age of forty. Next to lung cancer, breast cancer is the leading cause of cancer-related deaths among women. Incidence of this disease has risen steadily over the past decade—but this rising figure may be due to the more widespread use of screening mammographies.

A mammogram is a simple, noninvasive, minimally uncomfortable test. You are asked to undress from the waist up and stand within the confines of the machine. A technician will then position your breasts, one at a time, on a plate and will bring down a second plate on top of the breast. The best X-ray is taken from the most compression, which means the fit will be tight, just for a minute.

The second set of pictures is taken from the side. You will be asked to place your arm around the arm of the machine, and the technician will position your shoulder so that the lymph nodes under your arm as well as your breast tissue can be seen. She will then bring a plate across the entire side of your breast and underarm and then will roll and squeeze it into place. Larger breasted women may need two pictures per breast.

Here are some important points to keep in mind about your mammograms:

❒ A mammogram should be done at a facility with ACR (American College of Radiology) accreditation to ensure that the equipment and staff are top notch.

❒ If you're premenopausal, schedule your mammogram about a week after your period when your breasts are least tender.

❒ If you have breast implants, be sure to tell the technician so that she can adjust the machine accordingly.

❒ Make sure the technician notes any skin moles on your chart. This may help in reading the X-ray.

❒ Avoid using deodorant or talcum powder prior to your exam so that the X-ray will be clear.

❒ Your pictures should have a preliminary reading by a radiologist while you're still in the office, just to make sure that they're clear enough for an accurate reading. If they're not, you can have a second set taken.

❑ Your physician should get back to you with the results within ten days.

## Important Medical Alternatives to Care

After having been diagnosed and treated for breast cancer, you are more likely to contract it in the other breast, and therefore, vigilant attention must be paid to preventive care afterwards.

The most promising drug to come along for cancer prevention is *tamoxifen*, which suppresses cancer cells that depend on estrogen for continued growth. Unfortunately, the main ingredient in this medication, *taxol*, is derived from the yew tree, which is in short supply. This makes the drug expensive and environmentally unappealing as well. And an additional drawback is that there has been a slight increase in the incidence of uterine cancer in women who take this drug.

A great deal more research must be done before medical science is able to prevent a recurrence. The best medicine, therefore, is the simplest. Make sure that diet, exercise, and professional monitoring are part of your regular schedule.

## Mastectomy or Lumpectomy

Cancer can be devastating, and it can kill. If all preventive means haven't worked, the unfortunate truth may be that you might have to lose a breast, or both breasts, in order to save your life.

A controversy rages these days as to whether a lumpectomy is as effective a surgical tool. If the cancer is clearly delineated in one area of the breast, can't just that area be excised?

The studies on women who've had the entire breast removed and those who've just had a lump removed seem to indicate that they fare just about equally. Some women in each category experience a recurrence, and some don't. Although it seems a lot more appealing to remove the lump and keep the breast intact, a lumpectomy must be followed by a course of radiation, which is debilitating and time consuming. You must have these treatments daily for five or six weeks after surgery. Also, radiation can be carcinogenic in and of itself—the younger you are, the more chance that it may cause another cancer.

You and your physicians (you should have at least a second, and probably a third opinion prior to surgery) will have to make this difficult call. There are no easy answers.

Even if surgery is the option of choice, be assured that the good life can continue after the battle with breast cancer has been won. Consider the adventures of the following women.

Sara Hildebrand, a 61-year-old grandmother from Neenah, Wisconsin, pushed her way up inch by inch, foot by foot, to the summit of Aconcagua in Argentina. Over 23,000 feet high, only the Himalayas would be a greater challenge.

Along with Sara were 22-year-old Ashley Cox of Charlottesville, Va., and sixteen other brave women, all headed by 45-year-old Laura Evans of Ketchum, Idaho. What most of these women had in common was a victory of another kind—surviving breast cancer. The goal of this group, known as Expedition Inspiration, was to raise $2.3 million—$100 per foot of climb—for the Breast Cancer Fund, whose purpose is to finance research on breast cancer. Raising this money was an added bonus. The real challenge was accomplishing a major personal goal after the trauma of dealing with this dreaded disease.

## Cosmetic Surgery

Many women are dissatisfied with what nature gave them and want to change it. Although, in this day of high-tech, innovative procedures, anything is possible—any type of surgery has its drawbacks as well as its rewards. Read everything you can about breast surgery—pro and con—before you make your choice.

BREAST RECONSTRUCTION. After mastectomy, breast reconstruction is an excellent choice. Sometimes, the cosmetic surgeon can come in right after the surgical oncologist is finished, and you can have both operations concurrently. Although this is a long procedure (about seven hours on the table, under anesthesia), it saves a second operation and a second recuperation.

Because of the impact that cancer has on women's lives, breast reconstruction can be a life-saver. Women frequently say that they feel like "freaks" after a mastectomy, as though they have completely lost their femininity. Yet, they were unwilling or terrified live under the threat of a possible cancer recurrence several years down the line, so they had the operation. Having breasts restored to their bodies actually makes it easier to cope with the stress of cancer. And so it is a highly recommended procedure. Whatever tissue of the breast still remains is used in conjunction with an implant, usually silicone or saline covered with polyurethane.

BREAST AUGMENTATION. But other women who don't have cancer and haven't gone through a mastectomy may also opt for cosmetic surgery. Many women feel that they will look ten years younger if they take this road. This may be because they've always felt they were too small or too large, or have lost a great deal of weight (which changes the configuration and size of the breasts) and are now so self-conscious about their natural endowment that it seriously affects their daily life and feelings of attractiveness.

An incision is made either at the marginal shelf where the lower part of the breast attaches to the chest wall, around the lower border of the areola under the nipple, or in the armpit.

The surgeon then inserts an implant into the pocket formed by the incision, either inside or outside the pectoral muscle. The procedure takes an hour or two under general anesthesia, and the scar is usually well concealed after the healing process of a few months.

Up to thirty percent of women who undergo this surgery do not have a good outcome—the breast may harden and become painful, requiring a second operation to remove scar tissue or replace the implant. Up to ten percent of those who have breast augmentation experience nipple sensitivity, infection, or poor healing of the scars.

ARE IMPLANTS SAFE—AND ARE THEY FOR YOU? Unfortunately, breast reconstruction and augmentation surgery is not without some significant drawbacks. Scores of women who underwent these procedures were horrified to learn that the silicone implants hadn't been adequately tested before they came on the market. The incidence of *capsular contracture* (hardened breasts) and implants rupturing inside the body was startling enough to cause Dow Chemical Company to offer millions of dollars in settlement to women who had been harmed by this surgery.

The Food and Drug Administration ruled that silicone gel implants could be used only for medically required surgery and not solely for cosmetic reasons. The silicone implants can cause inaccurate mammogram readings, they may interfere with breastfeeding, and there is an increased risk of autoimmune disease, such as rheumatoid arthritis or lupus. Other symptoms triggered by silicone usage are chronic fatigue, hair loss, chest rashes, and an inability to swallow.

There are still proponents of silicone implants. However more physicians are using saline (salt water) implants these days, and for good reason. Many experts have denounced the silicone gel implants as being a guaranteed source of life-long problems. There are so many documented cases of moving and shifting implants which result in mismatched breasts and allergic reactions. At least one brand of implant has been associated with an increased incidence of cancer in animal studies. And the implants don't last a lifetime. At one point or another, they may have to be replaced, requiring more surgery and the risk of rupture during removal.

My own feeling is that you should avoid this surgery at all costs, or insist on saline implants if you do choose to have it. If the reason you want the surgery is that you believe you will look younger and sexier with bigger breasts, invest in some good, supportive lingerie that will do the same thing for your contour as implants. Most good relationships evolve from an appreciation of the uniqueness of the other person—their character, sense of humor, intellect, sense of compassion, as well as their looks. Bigger is *not* always better.

BREAST REDUCTION. Many women feel that the size of their large breasts severely impedes them from conducting active, normal lives. Sleeping is uncomfortable, jogging and other sports can be painful, and proper support bras are hard to find and tend to be uncomfortable. Then, too, when you turn heads all the time, you're not always sure if you should consider those stares as admiring or humiliating.

In order to reduce the size of the breast, an incision is made from the nipple down to the marginal shelf under the breast and then along the margin. Excess tissue is removed, and the nipple is repositioned.

This is major surgery, and can result in a good deal of scarring. The breasts may not be even, and the operation may interfere with breastfeeding. Diabetes and obesity increase the risks of this type of surgery.

BREAST LIFTS. For women who have borne and nursed many children or have lost a lot of weight, the *mastoplexy* may be a solution. This surgery lifts sagging tissue and restores the shape of the breast.

The surgery is similar to that for breast reduction, but the incisions are made differently. Two flaps of skin are cut open, from the areola down to the marginal shelf, and then a third cut is made at the shelf cutting away from the descending incisions. The excess tissue is removed and the remaining skin is sewn together in the shape of an anchor.

The scars hopefully fade with time, and generally, nipple sensitivity remains. A supportive bra should be worn day and night for four to six months after this procedure.

Will you be happier, sexier, younger-looking after cosmetic surgery? This is anyone's guess. I would say that you must know yourself well to be able to say how the operation will affect you. If you are a person who looks at the positive side of life, and know that changing your appearance will make a difference, then the chances are that surgery is a good idea. But if you are always criticizing yourself, if nothing is ever really good for you, then breast surgery will simply be an expensive, uncomfortable, possibly risky venture.

What we're aiming for is better care of our reproductive system to ensure a longer life. Let's think about the other organs in your system—your uterus, ovaries, and vagina, and see how they fit into your longevity picture.

## REPRODUCTIVE HEALTH AS YOU AGE

One of the most exciting things about living at the end of the twentieth century is that we have so many new possibilities. Our reproductive health is of key importance the longer we live, because it can help us retain our youthful interests, and also because it mirrors the health of the body in general. When we get these organs into excellent shape, we should have no trouble feeling as though we've gained a decade of life and gained a better sense of ourselves.

## Pregnancy over Thirty-Five

Only a few decades ago, a woman's reproductive life was over by the time she hit 35. But today, thanks to the advent of high-tech interventions and different lifestyles, women have the option to continue bearing children into their fifties. You can have a career, develop your personal skills, become a mature individual, and then become a mother, if you so choose. And many more mature mothers have said that having a baby or toddler around definitely gave them an extra lease on life. There is no way to feel elderly when you're rolling around on the floor or swinging from the branches with your kids.

## Fertility over Thirty-Five

About 10 percent of the reproductive-age population in the United States (approximately 5.3 million American women plus their partners) are infertile. This means that they cannot conceive a child within a twelve-month period of having unprotected sex. There are a number of factors that contribute to this problem—prior illnesses, the use of recreational drugs, a chemical imcompatibility between male and female partners—but the biggest one is age. The older you are, the fewer viable eggs you have left in your ovaries. Fertility peaks around age 30 in women and declines rapidly in the early 40s when ovulation becomes less regular. At this point in her life, she has a one in five chance of conceiving without any intervention.

1. *Charting temperature and mucus.* If you've been trying to get pregnant without success, you should first keep a temperature and mucous chart. Take your temperature first thing in the morning, before getting out of bed. The temperature will be low between your menses and ovulation stages and then will rise sharply as you ovulate and progesterone surges in your body. It will stay high for the next two weeks or until your period.

Your mucous is fertile just before your temperature goes up. For several days before the rise in your temperature, your mucous will have a creamy, pasty texture and be somewhat "stretchy" when you move it between your fingers. You are fertile as long as you have this stretchy mucous and for the three "dry" days after your temperature rises.

While you are keeping your charts, your partner should have a sperm test. He will be asked to produce a sample by masturbating into a specimen cup at the doctor's office; the sample will be checked for volume, mobility, and structural viability. The doctor will want to determine whether enough of these sperm will be able to make the journey up the vagina past the cervix and into the uterus to fertilize an egg.

2. *Medical work-up.* If six months of faithful charting and unprotected intercourse haven't worked, you will probably want to think about starting a medical work-up. This can be a very long and painstaking procedure, and many couples find that it interferes with their sex life, their relationship with each other and with their families, and that it may actually kill their desire to have a child. Years of testing, medication, and scheduled sex can wear you down more than childlessness. Yet there are so many wonderful children out there who need a home and are eligible for adoption.

If you do choose the medical route, here's a sampling of what to expect. You'll have blood tests for hormone levels, a radioisotope dye will be injected into your reproductive system to be sure the fallopian tubes are open, you'll have an X-ray of the uterus and fallopian tubes, ultrasound of the pelvic cavity, and you'll have to go to the hospital for a laparoscopic exploration of the pelvic cavity. Any abnormal findings, of course, would lead to separate treatments to correct whatever condition you might have.

3. *Medication.* If your infertility stems from ovulation problems, your doctor will probably start you on a course of medication. Approximately one-third to one-half of all infertile women have difficulty ovulating or don't ovulate at the right time for optimum fertilization, and these drugs can temporarily correct the various problems so that an egg can be released and rendezvous with a sperm in order to conceive a baby.

*Clomid (clomiphene citrate)* is the most commonly used to stimulate ovulation in women who have infrequent periods and long cycles. It's taken orally for five days of your cycle and costs about eight dollars per pill. When taken appropriately, it causes ovulation in 80 to 90 percent of women; about half of these will achieve a pregnancy within the first six treatment cycles. This drug does, however, produce twins in ten percent of all users. The miscarriage rate has been reported to be as high as 26 percent.

There are a variety of side effects to Clomid, including hot flashes, breast tenderness, nausea, headaches and insomnia. Overstimulation of the ovaries can result in ovarian cysts which can cause pelvic discomfort.

*Pergonal (human menopausal gonadatropin)* is the second most popular fertility drug, although it is very expensive and the number of office visits to your doctor bump the fees up even higher. It is administered by injection for seven to twelve days of your cycle, and contains equal parts of the two pituitary hormones, FSH and LH. During your course of treatment, your estrogen levels are monitored carefully to be sure you're getting the correct dosage. There can be severe complications resulting from this drug, including swollen, painful ovaries from being overstimulated. Ninety percent of users will ovulate following this treatment, and 20 to 60 percent will conceive on this drug. The incidence of multiple births is about 20 percent. This hormone is also used to develop multiple follicles (containing multiple eggs) for IVF or GIFT (see below).

*Parlodel (bromocriptine)* is used for women who have elevated levels of prolactin, a pituitary hormone in the brain that is generally secreted during breastfeeding. Elevated levels may stop the normal ovulatory cycle, however, Parlodel reduces the amount of prolactin released by the pituitary into the bloodstream. In 80 percent of patients treated with this drug, which is taken orally, normal menses occur in about six weeks. Approximately 85 percent of those treated will ovulate and can become pregnant if no other sources of infertility exist. However, as soon as the drug is discontinued, prolactin rises again and menses may cease. There are few side-effects to this medication, although some patients experience nausea, headache, constipation, low blood pressure when standing up too fast, and nasal stuffiness. Some studies report that the success rate for conception is higher than with other fertility drugs.

4. *Surgical repair.* If examination has proved that problems with your reproductive organs are contributing to your infertility, corrective surgery may be necessary. You may have an *ovarian wedge section,* to restore the function of diseased ovaries; *tubal insufflation,* to clear any blockage in the fallopian tubes; or *uterine suspension,* to move the uterus to a more receptive position so that conception will be easier.

5. *Assisted reproduction technologies (art).* If all previous methods have failed, you may choose ART. The possibilities are artificial insemination, in vitro fertilization detailed in the following, or gamete intrafallopian transfer. There are 40,000 babies born in this country as a result of these different technologies.

AI (ARTIFICIAL INSEMINATION). A sperm sample (either your husband's or that of an anonymous donor through a sperm bank) is introduced into your vagina, near the cervix, during one of the fertile days of your cycle after your ovaries have been stimulated with Pergonal. It may take several sessions (over four to six months) to achieve a pregnancy, but some success rates are as high as 70 to 80 percent.

Your husband's sperm is suitable for insemination if his sperm count is greater than 20 million sperm per cubic centimeter and more than 50 percent of the ejaculate has good motility forward.

If you choose donor insemination, you must be certain that:

1. The sperm you're using has been frozen for six months following which the donor was tested for AIDS, chlamydia, genital herpes, gonorrhea, and hepatitis B.

2. Your donor has not fathered more than ten offspring, to avoid problems of intermarriage.

3. Your sperm donor is younger than 40, to minimize the danger of any age-related damage to his sperm.

IVF (IN VITRO FERTILIZATION). This type of ART is for the woman who has one functional ovary, even if she has damaged or blocked fallopian tubes. If you select IVF, you are given Pergonal as well as the hormone, GnRH, so that you will mature several ova at once. These eggs are removed from your ovary during a laparoscopy or retrieved through the vagina during an ultrasound treatment. The ova are placed in a glass dish where they are fertilized by your husband's or a donor's sperm. If fertilization does occur, the ova are introduced into your uterus with a catheter and you are given progesterone to help support the resulting pregnancy. Usually, two to four embryos are transferred per cycle with the hope that one will survive and grow to term.

One cycle of IVF currently costs about $7,800, and typically, couples must try for about five to six months before achieving a pregnancy.

GIFT (GAMETE INTRAFALLOPIAN TRANSFER). This is a process where the ova and sperm are joined in the glass dish, but are immediately reintroduced into your body at the opening of your fallopian tube. In this way, fertilization can occur in the body as it might have naturally.

ART WITH DONOR EGGS. For the woman over 35 who may not have many viable eggs left in her ovaries, there is always the possibility of using someone else's ova. The egg donor can be a close relative (so that you can get a close genetic match), or an anonymous donor. During this procedure, the eggs are fertilized in vitro as described above and then inserted into the birth mother's uterus. This remarkable but very costly procedure can work even for women past menopause.

## Other Considerations in Pregnancy over Age Thirty-five

The aging process can't be stopped, so there are increased concerns with pregnancy in an older mother. The rates of miscarriage and birth defects are considerably higher. Women past 35 miscarry twice as often as younger women, but you can lower your risk by eating right; avoiding all drugs, alcohol, and caffeine; and staying away from environmental pollutants such as exposure to chemicals, tap water near industrial sites, and video display terminals.

If you are an older mother, or if you have a history of miscarriage, you may want to discuss progesterone supplementation with your medical doctor. Progesterone, which naturally supports a pregnancy, can be enhanced in the body, and is particularly effective if you have experienced luteal phase problems during your menstrual cycles.

Older parents-to-be are generally offered genetic counseling when they first decide to start trying to conceive. The reason is that the risk of chromosomal abnormalities rises dramatically from 1 in 500 in a 22-year-old mother to 1 in 192 at age 35. The risk for Down's syndrome is only 1 in 1500 for a 22-year-old mother, but by age 35, it's up to 1 in 378 births.

To be an informed older parent, there are several procedures that you may select in order to monitor the well-being of your child. The first, *amniocentesis*, involves taking a sample of the amniotic fluid from your uterus when you are from three to four months pregnant and testing it for chromosomal abnormalities. The second, *chorionic vilii sampling*, can be done in the first six weeks of your pregnancy. In this procedure, which does not give as much information as the amnio, a sampling is taken from the membrane at the mouth of the cervix.

Parents who feel that they would not be capable of raising a child with serious mental or physical impairment will probably want to have these procedures performed. However, there are risks involved. The amnio must be done when you are at the end of your first trimester and already anticipating parenthood. If the fetus is not in a good position, the puncture may not yield enough fluid for the test, or may do some physical damage to the growing baby. Then, too, neither amniocentesis nor chorionic sampling gives a complete picture of possible genetic or developmental problems.

On the plus side, however, if you are truly motivated to go through a pregnancy and birth at this stage of your life, you are probably a person who is naturally concerned with her health and who has been taking good care of both body and mind for years. It's possible that you might be in better shape than many women far younger than you—and mature and experienced enough to be a really good parent.

### Natural Strategies to Improve Your Fertility

1. Stop smoking, drinking alcohol or caffeine, or using recreational drugs.

2. Start a regular stress reduction program. This might be a great time to start meditating or practicing yoga or tai chi chuan.

3. Exercise daily. This might be a brisk walk, a daily swim, or regular visits to a health club.

4. Eat right, and be sure to increase your supplementation of folic acid. A deficiency of it has been shown to produce neural tube defects such as spina bifida. You should also be taking vitamins C and E, and zinc.

## Minimizing Your Risk of Cancers of the Reproductive System

If you're seeing a gynecologist once a year, he or she will be checking you for the possibility of any problems with your uterus, cervix, fallopian tubes, and ovaries. You can practice good preventive healthcare if you know your risks.

UTERINE, ENDOMETRIAL AND CERVICAL CANCER. Over 10,000 women die from these cancers each year, yet they are the easiest to detect. They are also the easiest to cure completely if caught in time, because they are slow growers.

Endometrial cancer is the most common gynecologic cancer in the United States and one of the six leading causes of cancer deaths in women. Cervical cancer (cancer of the neck of the uterus) is the fourth most common cancer of women, and 60,000 women a year are diagnosed with it. The best preventive treatment, again, is awareness of what your body is like when it's well so that you can tell if anything has changed.

1. *Have a yearly exam and Pap smear.* This is the best check for cervical abnormalities. The affected area can be treated by cauterizing or freezing.

2. *Be alert to dysfunctional bleeding.* If you're bleeding in between periods or after your menopause, tell your physician, who may want to remove a small sample of tissue from your uterine lining (an endometrial biopsy). If the tissue is hyperplastic (abnormally overgrown), or if bleeding continues, your doctor may do a D&C (dilation and curettage) where the entire endometrium (the lining of the uterus) is scraped away. This treatment may take care of the bleeding problem and eliminate the possibility that a cancer might develop.

3. *Stop smoking.* Nicotine and tars are poisons to your system and deprive all your cells of sufficient oxygen.

4. *Lose weight* if you are more than 20 percent over your ideal weight range.

5. *Lower your blood pressure.* Exercising and starting a dedicated stress management program will do more for you than medication in most cases, as will balancing the amounts of sodium and potassium in your diet (see Chapter Nine).

6. *Always practice safe sex.* Using a condom each and every time is essential if you are not in a mutually monogamous relationship.

It's clear that smoking, obesity, unsafe sex, and high blood pressure are risk factors for uterine, endometrial, and cervical cancer. Others that you should be aware of are:

1. Diabetes

2. Being of African-American descent

3. Family history of uterine cancer

4. History of ovarian tumor

5. History of endometrial hyperplasia (a thickening of the uterine lining)

6. History of sexually transmitted diseases such as chlamydia, genital warts, gonorrhea or syphilis.

7. Unmonitored estrogen replacement therapy without a progestin to slough off the lining of the uterus.

8. Over age 50

9. Lack of routine gynecological care and yearly pelvic exams

10. Never having used oral contraceptives, which balance the hormonal environment over time and protect against cancers of the uterus and ovaries.

OVARIAN CANCER. This silent but deadly illness claims over 13,000 lives a year. There are usually no warning signs, which prevents early detection. The best defense, however, in addition to routine pelvic exams, is long-term use of oral contraceptives or multiple pregnancies. The reason is that normal ovulation, which continally traumatizes the ovary, may result in the growth of abnormal cells, whereas having many babies or having your ovulation suppressed medically protects this delicate tissue.

You are most at risk for this disease if:

1. You've never given birth.

2. You don't have routine pelvic exams.

3. You have a family history of ovarian cancer or a personal history of breast cancer.

4. You are of African-American descent.

5. You've never taken oral contraceptives.

6. You completed menopause before age 50.

7. You are over age 60.

It's important to remember that your reproductive system doesn't exist in isolation—it's a part of your total being. By following the guidelines in other chapters in this book, you'll be boosting your immune system and keeping your entire body as youthful as possible. This can't help but improve your possibility of having a baby if you so wish. It will also lower your probability of developing a cancer, and enhance your sexuality.

Understanding the benefits—physical, mental, emotional and spiritual—of sexual and reproductive health can be an important component in adding ten years to your life.

# KEEPING
## YOUR BONES YOUNG

CHAPTER 7

$W$e have plenty of expressions that mean a person is weak, and they all revolve around our bones: "She hasn't got a leg to stand on"; or "She's just spineless." The real truth of the matter is that as we age, our skeleton does too, and if we haven't got a strong set of legs or hips or a back we can truly rely on, we may be courting trouble.

Estrogen helps to retain the calcium in the bone tissue instead of letting it leach out into the bloodstream. As women reach menopause, and their estrogen levels drop, it becomes increasingly difficult to keep the same bone mass and density they had when they were younger.

## WHAT YOU NEED TO KNOW ABOUT
## OSTEOPOROSIS

Osteoporosis, which means "porous bones," is the silent killer of women over 50. It causes over 1.3 million fractures a year in people over 45. More significantly, this condition affects one third to one half of all postmenopausal women. It can result in loss of height, a stooped posture or humpback, easily fractured bones, and a great deal of pain. Osteoporosis has social and emotional consequences

183

that are far reaching: A woman who breaks her hip and is confined to a walker or wheelchair when it doesn't heal properly may be unable to go out to see friends, or shop, or even get herself to the kitchen to make a cup of soup. The terrible isolation and dysfunction may cause her to become seriously depressed and unable to care for herself.

Although men can be afflicted with this condition, they typically start out with bigger, heavier bones, and of course, they aren't dependent on estrogen, but rather on testosterone for healthy bone growth. And women typically live six and a half years longer than men in our society, which means they have that many more years to become susceptible to this disease.

Osteoporosis is, in reality, a childhood condition that manifests itself in the geriatric population. Lack of exercise and calcium in the diet during childhood takes its toll many decades later. For this reason, it's urgent that all women know how to take care of their bones when they're young so that they'll be in the best shape possible when they're older.

## How the Bone Remodeling Process Changes as We Age

Bone is a living, growing tissue that is always changing, reacting to chemical, electrical and mechanical stimuli inside and outside the body. When we're younger, most of our bone has a 10 percent yearly turnover rate—new tissue is always replacing or remodeling the old tissue.

But after 35, this process doesn't work as well as we'd like. The old bone cells are removed, but new ones may not fill in the spaces completely. Or the quality of new bone may not be as strong as the former, younger bone. The outside frame of the skeleton, the white shiny tissue called *cortical bone*, often remains as it is. However, the inside structure, the *trabecular bone*, gets thinner until there isn't enough of it to support the outside shell. This inner matrix, shot through with capillaries, blood vessels, and marrow, at first looks regular in texture. But as time wears the body down, the cells that take bone away are more active than the ones that build it up. The inside of bone starts to look like a cyclone fence with lots of broken wires. And it's at this point that fractures may begin.

Hormones play a big role in your osteoporosis picture. Estrogen loss at menopause is thought to be one of the biggest factors in the development of this condition, since estrogen is greatly responsible for keeping calcium within the bone tissue. The adrenal glands are also important. Among other hormones, they produce a stress hormone called *cortisol*, which affects glucose and amino acid metabolism. Excess cortisol also seems to block the appropriate immune response if something goes wrong in the body. The thyroid gland produces *thyroxine*, which in large quantity can increase the amount of calcium secreted in the urine and can stimulate too much bone resorption. The *parathyroids* produce a hormone that reduces the amount of vitamin D in the body, which also lowers calcium supply to the bones.

# RISK FACTORS FOR OSTEOPOROSIS

There are certain factors you cannot change that predispose you to osteoporosis. There are other factors you can alter completely, thereby reducing your overall risk.

## Factors You Can't Change

1. *Sex*. Being female puts you at higher risk because your bones are smaller and lighter to begin with.

2. *Age*. Being past menopause puts you at higher risk because of your declining supply of estrogen to keep calcium in the bone.

3. *Family background*. If your mother or grandmother had this condition, and you are built like them, there's a good chance that you also have a predisposition to it.

4. *Race*. Being Caucasian or Asian puts you at greater risk. African-American and Hispanic women tend to have heavier bones.

5. *Fair complexion, small frame*. No one is certain why fair skin and hair is a risk factor for osteoporosis. But smaller bones means that even at your peak for bone mass, which is 35, you are at a disadvantage, which will become more significant as your bone mass and density decrease over the years.

## Factors You Can Change

1. *Smoking*. There is no question that cigarettes are a risk factor, since smokers go through menopause an average of five years earlier than nonsmokers. This means their estrogen supply is diminished sooner. Smoking also interferes with the formation of new bone tissue.

2. *Diet*. You are at higher risk if you don't have enough dietary calcium and vitamin D, and if you consume lots of caffeine and soft drinks. Caffeine inhibits bone formation and increases the amount of calcium lost in your urine. Soft drinks contain phosphates which bind to calcium so that it is difficult to metabolize.

3. *Lack of weight-bearing exercise*. Physical inactivity is a huge risk factor, since your bones need to be stressed by working against gravity in order to grow stronger. If you spent 36 weeks in bed after being in a car accident, for example, that would be equivalent to ten years of aging on your bones. Think of what this means if you've been a couch potato most of your life.

4. *Thinness and dieting*. If you're thin, you have fewer fat cells in your body. But after menopause, the fat cells of your body use a particular hormone called *androstenedione* and convert it into a weaker variety of estrogen called *estrone*. The fewer fat cells, the less estrone and the less protection to your bones. Yo-yo dieting, where you lose a great many pounds and then put them on again, changes the balance of hormones and enzymes in your body and wreaks havoc with bone formation.

5. *Childlessness or long lactation period*. Bone density increases during pregnancy. This is partly due to hormonal changes in the body to supply additional support to the baby. If you never have the experience of carrying a child to term, your bones don't have the opportunity to gain excess bone tissue.

If you do bear children, but nurse them longer than a year each, you are depleting your own body of calcium in order to supply it to your child.

6. *Oophorectomized*. If you have had both ovaries removed because they were damaged or cancerous, you no longer produce estrogen, which protects your bones. (Even if one ovary can be saved, you retain a good deal of your hormonal protection against osteoporosis and heart disease.)

As you can see, osteoporosis is a condition that can be changed and improved. Take the following test, which will give you a barometer on your own risk factors. Circle the answer that applies to you for each item.

## OSTEOPOROSIS SENSITIVITY TEST

| | 1 | 2 | 3 | 4 | 5 |
|---|---|---|---|---|---|
| 1. Do you regularly eat red meat? | No | | ? | | Yes |
| 2. Do you eat less than you should due to bulimia or similar eating disorder? | No | | ? | | Yes |
| 3. Are you a vegetarian? | No | | ? | | Yes |
| 4. Do you usually add salt to your food? | No | | ? | | Yes |
| 5. How many cups of caffeine do you drink daily? | 0 | 1-2 | 3-4 | 5-6 | >6 |
| 6. Do you avoid milk and other dairy products? | No | | ? | | Yes |
| 7. How many packs of cigarettes do you smoke? | 0 | $1/2$ | 1 | $1/2$ | >2 |
| 8. How many times a week do you exercise? | 3 | 7 | 2 | 1 | 0 |
| 9. Do you have any thyroid problems? | Yes | | No | | |
| 10. What is your age? | 40 | 50 | 60 | 70 | 80 |
| 11. How many pounds less than average do you weigh for your height? | None | | 10 | | 20 |
| 12. Are you African, native American, East Indian or Polynesian descent? | Yes | | mixed | | No |
| 13. Do you have fair skin and complexion? | No | | ? | | Yes |
| 14. Are you small-boned? | No | | ? | | Yes |
| 15. Are you allergic to milk and dairy products? | No | | ? | | Yes |
| 16. Have you ever given birth? | Yes | | No | | |
| 17. Did you breast-feed any children? | No | | 2 or more | | 1 |
| 18. Have you gone through menopause before age 45? | No | | | | Yes |
| 19. Have you had your ovaries removed? | No | | | | Yes |
| 20. Is there a family history of osteoporosis or other bone disease? | No | | ? | | Yes |

When you've finished, assign the number 1 through 5 (at the top of each row) to your response. For example, if you smoke 1 pack a day, assign the number "3." If you're 50 years of age, assign the number "2," and so on. Then add up all the assigned numbers.

If your score is 20-39, you're in great shape. If your score is 40-69, you might consider changing some of your lifestyle habits, as described in this chapter. If your score is over 70, then this chapter is very important to you—have an osteoporosis work-up by your physician, and give strong consideration to beginning HRT.

Item 8 may confuse you, so let me explain. There's no doubt that exercise is beneficial, but exercising every other day is slightly better than exercising daily as far as bone health is concerned. The difference is small, though. Exercising every day is slightly better than exercising twice a week but not as good as exercising 3 times a week. In other words, too much of anything is not necessarily the best.

## CALCIUM IN YOUR DIET AND IN YOUR BONES

Calcium is the prime mineral component of your bones. But the body constantly needs a fresh supply of dietary calcium to keep bones uniformly strong.

A calcium-rich diet is essential, and in addition to this vital mineral the diet should be low in saturated fats, low in sugar and salt, high in fiber, and high in complex carbohydrates. Remember that calcium isn't just found in dairy products, although that's what most people think of when they think of calcium. In fact, it's much better to ingest this mineral from green leafy vegetables like kale and collard greens, and fish with bones like mackerel and salmon. You can also select calcium-enriched orange juice and oatmeal. You'll keep your diet lower in fat if you don't rely on dairy for your calcium.

One reason to avoid dairy is because of its high fat content. But if you can tolerate skim milk, you can get a good deal of your calcium this way. Fat interferes with calcium absorption, which is why skim milk is beneficial in an osteoporosis prevention diet.

In addition to the following osteoporosis-prevention diet, you should be taking the vitamins I recommend in Chapter Two.

# DR. RYBACK'S OSTEOPOROSIS PREVENTION DIET

## Breakfast

1 cup orange or grapefruit juice *or* 1 fruit

1 serving oatmeal or oat bran cereal with skim milk, sprinkled with raisins, berries or sliced banana

1 cup decaffeinated coffee with milk or herb tea

*Twice a week, add:*

1 slice whole wheat toast *or* 1 wheat or raisin English muffin covered with low-fat cheese

## Lunch

1 turkey *or* water-packed tuna sandwich on whole wheat bread made with lettuce and tomato

1 cup skim milk *or* fat-free yogurt *or* 10 oz. cream of tomato soup made with skim milk

1 fruit

1 glass iced herbal tea

*Three times a week, replace sandwich with:*

1 vegetarian casserole or stir-fry of your choice, including kale, collard greens, or turnips

## Mlidafternoon Snack

1 cup milkshake made by blending $1/2$ cup skim milk *or* nonfat yogurt with fruit

## Dinner

1 serving baked filet of sole *or* broiled whitefish *or* poached salmon *or* broiled perch *or* baked skinless chicken

1 serving each of two fresh green or yellow vegetables.

*Three times a week, one of your vegetables should be a baked or boiled potato with skin*

1 whole wheat roll

1 fresh fruit

1 cup skim milk or fat-free yogurt

1 cup decaffeinated coffee or herb tea

*Twice a week, replace fish or chicken dish with:*

1 serving of pasta or casserole of your choice

## Evening Snack

1 cup skim milk

1 slice angel food cake covered with berries *or* 8 ginger snap cookies *or* 1 cup airpopped popcorn.

Unfortunately, even if you follow my diet to the letter, you probably can't get all the calcium you need. As we age, our gut absorbs less, and it becomes harder to retain the nutrients, vitamins, and minerals we ingest. Most women who eat a traditional American diet are only getting 400 to 500 mg. of calcium per day, unless they are big milk drinkers. And as they get older, they aren't absorbing nearly that much from the foods they eat.

Older women tend to drink less milk and eat less food. They also tend to get out less in the sunlight, which decreases the amount of Vitamin D they get daily. This vitamin works together with calcium to produce good bone mass and density. Older women also tend to take a good many medications, and many drugs interfere with calcium absorption.

This is the reason that supplementation is essential. You can take calcium tablets which are usually packaged with magnesium or Vitamin D. Some also contain a mineral called *boron*, which assists in better absorption. You can also take Tums or other antacids without aluminum in them. Although the FDA recommends a daily allowance of 800 mg. for most people, it's far too low to prevent osteoporosis. Before menopause, all women should be consuming 1,000 mg. a day of calcium. If you're pregnant or nursing, you need about 1,500 mg. a day, which is what you'll need after menopause.

You don't need to worry about overdosing on this amount of calcium unless you have a family or personal history of kidney stones or kidney infection. In that case, you must have a doctor's recommendation to decide what is appropriate for you. You should never exceed 3,000 mg. per day, because this much calcium might cause a zinc deficiency.

## AEROBIC FITNESS: LET GRAVITY HELP YOUR BONES

In the early 1960s, NASA sent astronauts into space for several days and measured the carpal bones in their fingers when they returned. All of the astronauts had lost bone mass during this brief period of time. The reason? Although they exercised and rode a stationary bike each day, they had no gravity to work against. During the next flight, the amount of calcium in their food was tripled, and the result was that none of them lost any bone tissue.

You have to work these bones hard throughout your life if you don't want them to start getting fragile after menopause. So although swimming is wonderful exercise, it isn't weight-bearing. Your body is carried by the water, and your bones aren't stressed. Walking, on the other hand, is good osteoporosis prevention.

In a study following 169 healthy women aged 35 to 62 over two years, it was discovered that aerobic fitness was important (among other factors) in preventing bone loss associated with osteoporosis. After a five-month program of arm exercises practiced three times a week, a group of postmenopausal women had increased their bone density, whereas the control group, who did no exercise, had lost density.

Exercise is also vital in terms of teaching you good alignment, balance, and coordination. If you stand firmly on your feet, and have good reflexes, you are less likely to trip and fall and possibly fracture a bone. Exercise also tones and shapes the muscles around bone, keeping the whole structure healthier.

The following is a list of possible regimens you can start to keep your bones in good shape. All you need in most cases is a good pair of shoes. You also should have a checkup so that your physician can give you the green light to begin an exercise program. If you already have osteoporosis, all of the following exercises may be too strenuous for you, and you will need a custom-designed program from an orthopedist or physical therapist.

It's important to make a commitment to your exercise program and to stick with it. Daily or every other day is next best, and three times a week is really minimal. It doesn't take long—perhaps half an hour—and it will give such a lift to your spirits that you'll derive a lot more out of it than just healthy bones. Of course, everything in moderation is the key—you don't want to become fanatic about this regimen because overexercising can put your body into a crisis mode as the proportion of lean body mass to fat changes dramatically. Premenopausal women who have no fat on their body are in danger of stopping their menstrual cycle, which is bad for the bones because estrogen supplies might be depleted.

## OSTEOPOROSIS-PREVENTION AEROBIC ACTIVITIES

| | |
|---|---|
| walking | jogging |
| biking | roller blading |
| aerobic dance | ballroom/jazz/modern dance |
| martial arts | step-training |
| rowing | jumping rope |
| low-impact aerobics | racquet sports |

Whichever activity you select, be sure that it's something you want to do, and will stick to. The idea is to get to like exercise, to have fun, and to feel that it's not a chore but an integral part of your life. If you're a people person, join a gym so that you can meet others, or go mall-walking. If you enjoy the solitude of nature, set your alarm half an hour early and enjoy watching the sun come up as you exercise.

You should also set a goal for yourself. Start slowly, and then, as your endurance and fitness level goes up, you can increase the intensity and duration of your regimen. Walkers, for example, might start with two miles over a half-hour and build up to three miles in 45 minutes. Joggers could reach for a goal of three miles in 30 minutes if they're under 60 and in 24 minutes if they're under 50.

## OSTEOPOROSIS-PREVENTION NON-AEROBIC ACTIVITIES

stretching

weight training

yoga

tai chi chuan

Stretching can and should be done by everyone, and if you're a beginner at exercise, you might want to start with this activity and stick with it for a while before selecting anything aerobic. Stretching strengthens your muscles, increases your range of motion, and helps promote endurance and flexibility—all requirements for strong bones.

## OSTEOPOROSIS-PREVENTION STRETCHING.

1. *Spine stretch standing.* Stand with your back to the wall, feet comfortably apart and legs slightly bent. Tighten your belly muscles

so that you bring your waist as close to the wall as possible. Hold for five seconds, then relax. Repeat ten times.

2. *Spine stretch prone.* Lie on your back, knees bent, feet flat on the floor, with small pillows under your head and the small of your back. Now contract your back, tightening your stomach muscles, so that your waist touches the pillow. Hold for five seconds, relax and repeat ten times.

3. *Cat stretch.* On your hands and knees, drop your head forward as you arch your back and tilt your pelvis under. Hold for five seconds, relax. Repeat five to ten times.

4. *Shoulder shrug.* Sit comfortably in a straight-backed chair or on a bench. Shrug your shoulders and bring them up as high as you can toward your ears, then let them relax downward. Next, bring your shoulders backward, pulling your shoulders back as though you were trying to pinch your shoulder blades together. Relax. Repeat this sequence five to ten times.

5. *Long muscle stretch.* Stand with your back to the wall, flattening your body against it. Raise your right arm and right heel at the same time and reach for the ceiling. Come back to center. Now stretch the left arm and left heel. Alternate side to side five times.

6. *Knee and hip stretch.* Lie on your back and pull both knees to your chest, wrapping your arms around them. Hold for a count of five and relax. Repeat ten times.

7. *Back stretch.* Sit on the floor with legs crossed, tailor style. Starting with your hands at your side, crawl your fingers behind you, letting your back arch. Then walk your hands back to center. Next, crawl your fingers forward as far as you can go in front of you. Walk your hands back to center. Repeat five times. Be sure you do equal numbers of flexing and extending exercises for your back.

Lifting weights is a wonderful activity for women, who typically don't have as much upper body strength as men. A recent study of fifty frail, elderly nursing home residents, some older than 90, surveyed the effects of hip and knee resistance exercises. In just ten weeks, exercising three times a week, all of the participants had improved strength and increased muscle size. They also had better mobility and more spontaneous activity.

Working out with light weights (start with about 2 or 3 pounds in each hand) will slowly increase both your bone mass and density. After a month you can move to five-pound weights. You'll want to increase your repetitions as well, from five when you begin to ten in about a month.

### OSTEOPOROSIS-PREVENTION WEIGHT LIFTING

1. Lie on your back, knees bent, feet flat on the floor, arms extended holding the weights facing up to the ceiling. Keeping your arms straight, lift the weights up toward and above your chest so that they meet in the middle. Return arms to the floor. Repeat five times.

2. Start with your arms at your sides, hands turned toward your body. Bending your elbow, bring one weight at a time up to a vertical position. Return arms to the floor. Repeat five times.

3. Start with your arms at your sides, palms down. Lift each arm alternately to a vertical position. Return to the floor. Repeat five times.

4. *Overhead press*. Sit on a chair or bench with your knees apart and hold the weights at shoulder level, palms facing in toward your body. Alternately, raise each weight straight above your head and then slowly back down again. Do five repetitions. Then bring both weights up together and do five repetitions.

5. *Curls*. Stand up and let your hands hang by your sides, palms facing forward. Raise each weight alternately to your shoulders. Repeat five times. Then lift both arms together five times.

No matter what form of exercise you're doing, keep breathing fully! You want to get oxygen to every cell in your body, and you can't do that if you hold your breath. Remember to sink your weight, drop your shoulders, and inhale right from your belly (see Chapter Four on breathing).

## Bone Densitometry Testing

Regardless of all the preventive strategies you use, at some point you are going to have to find out exactly how your bones are adjusting to the aging process. Particularly if you have numerous risk factors for osteoporosis, it's important that you make the effort to get a bone screening so that you and your physician will know how to proceed.

Bone densitometry testing is an easy, effective way to learn whether or not you've lost bone, if you've lost an average amount or whether you are a fast bone loser—in which case it's advisable to start taking medication to prevent further damage. The test is available at most major medical centers, and in the offices of some orthopedists and endocrinologists. There are also dedicated osteoporosis centers around the country where you can have a screening.

Currently, this diagnostic test is not covered by third-party payers, and it will cost from $200 to $400, depending on where you live, to have your spine and hip assessed. But the test is well worth it, because it affords a great deal of information that's not available by any other means.

Your doctor will probably do some blood tests first, to measure red and white blood cell counts, as well as test for protein, calcium, phosphorus, parathyroid and thyroid hormone levels, and vitamin D levels. He or she will also give you a 24-hour urinary calcium and creatinine excretion test to determine how much calcium you lose in your urine. There are some new and very sensitive urine tests that can determine how quickly bone is being resorbed. These tests might be performed on an elderly woman who has just suffered several fractures, for instance.

All these tests are markers not only for what is happening in your body right now, but also for what may occur in the future. But the best measurement is the bone densitometry test.

Bone mineral density shows up as a radiographic picture on a computer screen. The scan shows bone mineral mass and density and gives readouts for each area scanned. These results are then compared to a compilation of measurements in the computer bank for women of reproductive age and then for postmenopausal women. In this way you are deemed a slow or fast bone loser. The machine also does an estimate of where your fracture threshhold lies.

Most women lose about 1 to 3 percent of their bone mass each year after menopause for the next seven or eight years, at which point they start to level off as their body achieves a new hormonal balance. But those who lose 5 to 6 percent of their bone mass are in serious danger of having fragile tissue that will fracture at the slightest bump. There are extremely high-risk women who break ribs just coughing or sneezing.

There are several different types of densitometry measurement:

1. *Single-photon absorptiometry* (SPA). This test uses a radioactive iso-tope passed through the forearm or wrist to determine the bone mass and density at that site.

2. *Dual-photon absorptiometry* (DPA). This test uses two isotopes from two different directions. It can examine thicker areas of the body such as the spine or hip and make an assessment about both cortical and trabecular bone.

3. *Dual-energy X-ray absorptiometry* (DEXA). This more sophisticated test uses an X-ray source. It is more accurate, takes less time and gives the patient a lower dosage of radiation.

4. *Quantitative computed tomography* (QCT). This test is basically a CT scan with specialized software. It can examine the whole body and can look at a cross-section of the vertebrae to assess the condition of trabecular bone. This is the most expensive of the tests, takes the greatest amount of time, and gives the highest dosage of radiation.

If your readings are in the normal to high-normal range, your doctor will use the densitometry tests as a barometer of how you're doing over time. If, for example, you start on a regimen of HRT after having this test, your doctor can check you in a year to see if your bone loss has slowed down. If you opt not to take medication, you can still be retested to see if you are stabilizing or losing more quickly.

By knowing where you stand, it will be easier for you to make important decisions about your healthcare so that you can keep your bones strong for another ten years, and another, and another.

## Hormone Replacement Therapy for Your Bones

If estrogen keeps the calcium in the bone and you lose estrogen at menopause, it would only be logical to consider replacing that hor-mone when you don't have enough of it. Hormone therapy—estro-gen alone for women who have no uterus or estrogen plus a prog-estin for those who do—has been found to be the most effective treatment for osteoporosis. Such therapy has been found to reduce fracture rates by 75 percent (vertebral) and 50 percent (hip). Long-term therapy is advised for this condition, and the statistics on ten to fifteen years of HRT are astounding: Ten years of HRT have been shown to reduce vertebral fracture by 90 *percent*.

Advocates say that for optimum protection, you should begin HRT at menopause and continue for the rest of your life. However, even women in their seventies and eighties can halt the bone loss that's occurred in prior decades. It's doubtful whether an octogenarian can actually increase bone mass and density, but maintaining what she's got and preventing further loss is certainly worthwhile.

HRT is not for every woman, even if she is at high risk for osteoporosis. See Chapter Five for a full discussion of the pros and cons of this treatment. It must be mentioned that long-term estrogen therapy does put you at higher risk for endometrial cancer. However, the risk of hip or vertebral fracture is far greater than contracting this particular cancer, which is slow-growing and can be easily caught as long as you are being monitored regularly by your physician.

It is quite a commitment to select a medical therapy that, to be effective, lasts about fifteen or twenty years. Remember that you can always change your mind, and wean yourself slowly off HRT, or you might consider other, nonhormonal therapies. The crucial point is that if you are informed, you can make choices. And these choices can certainly extend your life.

### Alternatives to HRT

Although there is no treatment that compares statistically with HRT for success in halting bone loss, there are other choices you can make.

*Calcitonin* is the best known of the nonhormonal treatments. This hormone, which blocks bone resorption, is present naturally in the blood, but when given in large doses, it acts as a drug. For women who cannot or choose not to take HRT, injectable calcitonin is available, and a nasal spray variety has just been recommended for approval by the FDA which should be available soon.

The experimental clinical trials with this drug have been very promising; sometimes, it is used in a combined treatment with *bisphosphonates* (see the following). In addition to slowing bone loss, calcitonin has the added plus of being a pain-killer. The analgesic effect should be even stronger in the nasal spray, since the drug will affect the brain through the olfactory glands.

*Didronel (etidronate)*, a bisphosphonate, is one of several drugs that have proved promising in clinical trials. Like estrogen, these drugs inhibit bone resorption by slowing down the action of the cells that eat away at old bone tissue. The clinical trials for these drugs have had mixed results, but apparently the fracture rate has not been promising enough to receive FDA approval. Didronel is FDA approved for the treatment of Paget's disease, and doctors are using it for osteoporosis because it's safe and increases bone density. But because the quality of new bone isn't strong, there is concern that patients will continue to fracture repeatedly on this medication.

Didronel is taken cyclically by mouth, two weeks on and two and a half months off. The cycling is to give the bone time to start remodeling on its own.

*Allendronate* is another bisphosphonate that seems slated for success, and may be on the market within the year. It, too, slows bone resorption and its fracture rate has been low in clinical trials. It is a more powerful drug than etidronate, and is therefore taken in a lower dosage. It doesn't have to be cycled, and the daily regimen of 5 mg. daily makes it easier to comply with. If it gains FDA approval, as it probably will, it will be a viable alternative to HRT in the treatment of osteoporosis.

Other medical approaches are in the research stage, and if you are a good candidate for an experimental program and live near a major city where such work may be under way, you could benefit from these innovative therapies. However, there are no promises. Currently, there is no cure for osteoporosis—all we can do is adopt preventive measures to slow bone loss.

Many alternative therapies, such as acupuncture, spinal manipulation and chiropractic, herbal and homeopathic remedies are useful to alleviate symptoms. Meditation can also reduce stress that may exacerbate stiffness and back pain. You may want to consult a practitioner in one of these complementary therapies after you have had your densitometry test and have had time to consult with your physician on your best course of treatment.

### Common Sense Bone-Saving Tips

There's a lot we can do every day in order to preserve our bones. Here are some useful tips to make sure you take the best possible care of your spine and hips:

### PERSONAL TIPS:

1. If you need eyeglasses, wear them. Too many needless accidents are caused by vanity.

2. Give up high heels and backless slippers. Wear good supportive shoes with rubber or leather soles.

3. Be careful about long coats and bathrobes, which can easily trip you up.

4. If you are ill or on medication, be aware that you are not as alert to your surroundings as you could be. The worst offenders are long-acting sedatives such as Valium, Librium, and Dalmane which are sometimes routinely prescribed for women who may or may not need them. Be wary of over-the-counter drugs that might distort your perception and balance.

5. Get a good firm mattress and a pillow that supports the curve of your neck.

6. Never sit in a couch, which is like a big trap—easy to get into, difficult to get out of. Instead, use a straight-back chair with arms.

7. Use a small pillow to support your lower back. Many excellent back support aids are available by mail order, in furniture stores or at chiropractic offices. It's a good idea to keep one support in the car and another at home.

8. Get up and stretch every twenty minutes. This is particularly important if you have a desk job.

9. When you get up, keep your knees lined up with your hips. Don't twist or turn around; don't splay your knees outward.

10. When you sit, either in a car or at a desk or computer terminal, make sure your knees are slightly higher than your hips.

11. When you get out of bed, prop yourself up on your arm first, then swing your hips around and raise up to a sitting position. With your feet flat on the floor, stand up.

### AROUND THE HOUSE:

1. Be sure the lighting is adequate on stairs and in hallways.

2. Tack down all electrical wires; put nonslip pads under your rugs.

3. Check to be sure the sidewalk outside your house is in good shape, with no broken or protruding pieces you might trip on.

4. If you need to open a window, stand close to it and bend your knees before you lift.

5. Don't shovel snow; pay a healthy young teenager to do it for you. If you absolutely have to do this chore yourself, invest in a back-saver shovel, with a crooked handle that makes lifting easier.

6. If you have to lift anything, bend your knees rather than your back. Carry the object close to your body at waist height. When carrying grocery or garbage bags, try and apportion the weight so you can carry equal amounts in both arms.

## What About Arthritis?

Your bones are affected by the aging process, but so are your joints—the places where bone meets bone. If the joints lose their lubrication and flexibility, you can develop arthritis. There are two main types of this condition that affect us as we grow older—*osteoarthritis* and *rheumatoid arthritis.*

*Osteoarthritis* is a degenerative joint disease that affects up to 50 percent of all women over age 45. It develops because of years of stress on the cartilage between the bones, resulting in the secretion of certain enzymes which destroy the adjoining tissue. As we get older, we have fewer and less effective proteins involved in repair and restoration of tissue, and so the affected joints become weak, and are often immobilized.

In addition, there is increasingly less lubrication around each joint, making it more difficult for the joints to move smoothly. The cartilage that protects the ends of each bone begins to wear away, leaving rough edges. It becomes more difficult for the joints in certain areas, such as the knees, hips, back, neck and hand, to stay flexible. As more cartilage chips away, the ends of the bones harden, and large bone spurs may grow, resulting in pain, deformity, and limited motion. Typically, the condition will affect either your right or left side, but not both.

*Rheumatoid arthritis* is a chronic inflammatory condition that affects the entire body, but is most prevalent at the synovial membranes between the bones at the joints. In this autoimmune disease, the body attacks itself. It literally cannot distinguish between the body's own elements and those of a foreign invader or pathogen. Generally the disease manifests itself in women between the ages of 20 and 40 and affects the wrists, ankles and knees. Unlike osteoarthritis, this condition affects both sides of the body equally. It's not known what triggers this form of arthritis, but there may be a genetic predisposition to it, as well as factors relating to nutrition and allergies.

*Arthritis Treatments.* The conventional therapy for both types of adult arthritis is two to four grams of aspirin a day. It's been found that a preventive dose of aspirin may protect you against heart attacks, as well (see Chapter Nine). Aspirin seems to work on pain by blocking synthesis of *prostaglandins*, which are a key part of the inflammatory process. Unfortunately, many women cannot tolerate this high a dosage because it may cause nausea, ringing in the ears, or temporary loss of hearing. In this case, they can take nonsteroidal, antiinflammatory drugs (NSAIDS) such as ibuprofen (Nuprin, Advil), Naprosyn, or Clinoril. These, however, can also upset your stomach, cause gastrointestinal bleeding, and dizziness.

There are many other arthritis treatments, such as *gold injections*, *antimalarial drugs*, and *penicillamines*. They may prevent flare-ups but all three have side effects and must be carefully monitored. Some physicians *treat* with *corticosteroids*, however these powerful drugs may in time destroy bone tissue.

So the best bet is the most natural approach. The following is my prescription to alleviate the suffering of arthritis pain.

## FOUR-STEP ARTHRITIS RELIEF PROGRAM

### 1. Diet

Too much weight on the joints creates a great deal of stress, so if you suffer from osteoarthritis, you should make sure that you remain in the correct weight range for your height. You can do this by following the Osteoporosis Prevention Diet ( p. 189) but also by cutting down on portion sizes.

In addition, you might try the following foods:

☐ Flavonoid fruits such as cherries and blueberries. Another help-ful fruit is fresh pineapple, which has been reported to alleviate arthritis pain, especially when combined with fresh ginger.

☐ Sulphur-containing foods such as onions, garlic, and Brussels sprouts which may reduce some of your swelling and alleviate pain.

☐ Cold-water fish, such as herring, mackerel, salmon and sar-dines. These contain omega-3 fatty acids which have a benefi-cial effect on inflammatory response. You can also take the fish oil itself—1.8 grams of *eicosapentaenoic acid* (EPA) daily.

☐ You may want to avoid foods in the nightshade family such as eggplant, potatoes, and tomatoes. In one study, eliminating these foods resulted in pain relief for 70 percent of the partici-pants tested.

If you have rheumatoid arthritis, you should be tested for food allergies. The most common culprits are wheat, corn, dairy products, red meat, and foods of the nightshade family.

## 2. Supplementation

Make sure you continue taking all the vitamins and minerals recom-mended for women (see Chapter Two). In addition, you should have the following:

For either type of arthritis:

1. Vitamin E, at least 400 IU daily.

2. Manganese, at least 5 mg. daily.

3. Pantothenic acid, 12.5 mg. daily has shown clinical improve-ment for arthritis sufferers.

For rheumatoid arthritis:

1. Zinc, 30 mg. daily for rheumatoid arthritis, preferably in the form of zinc picolinate or citrate.

2. Curcumin (Curcuma longa) is an antiinflammatory agent taken from the yellow pigment of turmeric. It should be taken in three daily dosages of 400 mg. each. This substance is usually combined with *bromelain*, which supports the effect of the curcumin.

For osteoarthritis:

1. Niacinamide, 900 mg. in three divided daily doses, can reduce the pain of osteoarthritis and improve the range of movement of affected joints. Be sure not to take the time-release form of this vitamin which can cause serious side effects. You should be monitored by a dietician or physician if you are taking this supplement.

2. Glucosamine sulfate, 500 mg. in three daily doses with meals, will reduce pain and inflammation better than aspirin or NSAIDS and offers long-term benefits. Glucosamine helps to stimulate the proteins necessary for joint repair and exerts a protective effect against destructive enzyme activity in the joints.

## 3. Exercise

If you're an arthritis sufferer, you are well aware that the pain of movement can keep you from maintaining a regular exercise schedule.

So your watchwords must be "slow and steady." As soon as you get up in the morning, work out the stiffness in your joints with gentle stretches, starting at your ankles and working your way up to your head. The more rotation you can get in each joint—your neck and jaw, hips and knees, shoulders, elbows, wrists, hands and fingers—the better. Yoga and tai chi chuan (discussed at length in Chapter Four), are probably the best forms of exercise for this condition you could select. Walking, swimming and cycling are also excellent activities.

## 4. No Smoking

This recommendation appears in every chapter with cause—smoking seriously affects every body organ. In the case of your bones and joints, it is particularly destructive because it interferes with adequate oxygen supply to your bloodstream and your capillaries are unable to nourish your bone tissue. Cigarettes also create more estrogen depletion in the body, and it's the estrogen that keeps the calcium in your bones and joints.

## Keeping Your "House" in Good Shape

Your bones and joints are more valuable parts of your anatomy than you could ever imagine because they provide structure and support for the delicate organs within. This means that if you intend to live for ten more years, you have to work from the outside in as well as from the inside out. Eat right, exercise, and get appropriate medical help when needed. Your bones and joints will thank you!

# AGE-PROOFING
## YOUR SKIN, HAIR, AND TEETH

## CHAPTER 8

Our society worships youth—the taut bodies, the flowing hair, the dewy skin. So naturally, we would all like to look ten years younger. Now, you can't turn back the clock, or stop it, but you can do a lot with motivation and creativity not just to live ten years longer but to grow more youthful looking at the same time. The younger you look, generally, the younger you feel and behave. In this chapter, we'll explore the changes that take place in your skin, hair and teeth, and offer suggestions on how to deal with them.

## YOUR SKIN AS YOU AGE

There are no miracles, no magic bullets for looking like a kid again. And as we age, we don't *want* to look childlike. What we're aiming for is a mature and natural image that complements the type of person we've become. The traumas of life have their effect on the face; however, there are ways to eliminate or reduce problems that prematurely age the skin, such as overexposure to the sun, lack of proper hygiene, poor diet, and substance abuse. We'll explore what women can and cannot do in order to age-proof their skin.

The skin is an organ that covers the entire body and is made up of two basic layers: the underlying *dermis* and the outer *epidermis*. They are made up (from inside out) of the *basal* or *germinative layer*, the *stratum spinosum*, the *stratum granulosum*, and the *stratum corneum*, or "horny" outer covering that we can see.

New skin cells are formed at the basal layer, starting off round and plump. Then they travel through the next three levels, getting older and flatter as they go, until they reach the outer, visible layer where they're prepared to be shed or scraped off. Dermatologists refer to the time it takes for this trip through the four layers as *transit time*, and the process of shedding as *desquamation*. If the cells are scraped off, as they are when we scrub our face, it's called *exfoliation*.

As you can see, the skin is a very active organ, hardly resting for a moment. But as you get older, the transit time slows down. The transit time of an 80-year-old woman is four to six weeks, as compared to that of a 20-year old, whose transit time is merely two to three weeks. The longer it takes the skin cells to get to the outer layer, the older and flatter are the cells when they get there. This is the reason that older skin doesn't have that shining, plumped-out glow.

Even as you enter your thirties, cell turnover begins to slow down, making your skin look somewhat duller. Your years of exposure to the sun begin to show up as fine furrows and laugh lines. Your skin sprouts small red "domes" known as *cherry angiomas*, and benign brown or grayish raised growths known as *seborrheic keratoses*.

## How Midlife Affects Your Skin

As you enter your forties, your skin begins to thin out ever so slightly, making it more susceptible to the harmful effects of the sun. Gravity starts to pull at your face and your skin loses some of its elasticity, causing noticeable sagging at the eyes and jowls. You may begin to see some occasional discoloration of your skin as well. The texture becomes drier in midlife, especially in cold, windy climates with less moisture in the air. Women who have gone through menopause may begin to grow a little facial hair, because of the decrease of estrogen in their system.

# AGE-PROOFING YOUR FACE

So how do you keep your skin from aging? Here are seven sure-fire ways to keep skin ten years younger.

1. Avoid overexposure to the sun
   - wear sunscreen—apply it generously and reapply as often as needed
   - wear a broad-brimmed sun hat
   - wear protective clothing
   - exercise outdoors primarily in the early morning or evening

2. Accelerate your skin's transit time
   - choose a gentle exfoliating technique (scrubs or cleansing grains)

3. Moisturize your skin
   - drink eight to ten glasses of water a day
   - apply moisturizers to your face

4. Avoid tobacco and excess alcohol

5. Feed your skin properly
   - Vitamins A, B, C and E are critical for youthful appearance.

6. Get enough sleep
   - During your seven or eight hours in bed, you secrete specific skin growth factors along with human growth hormone. These hormones speed up production of collagen, the protein responsible for elasticity and support of skin tissue, as well as a faster rate of exfoliation.

7. Consider these treatments which your doctor can prescribe or perform:
   - Retin-A
   - dermabrasion
   - chemical peel

## HOW TO PROTECT YOUR SKIN FROM THE SUN

The biggest key to retaining youthful skin is to keep it sun-free as much as possible. I shudder when I see people catching some rays with a hand-held reflector—it's like inviting the aging process to start even earlier. The price isn't paid for sunworshipping until years later, when wrinkled skin and liver spots become apparent.

Loss of smoothness is only one aspect of sun damage. Radiation-damaged skin shows *pigment variation* (light and dark patches or mottling), *thinning of the epidermis, yellowing, fine beading*, and *telangiectasia* (blood vessel enlargement) which is seen as *red lines, fanning*, or *branching*. Sunburn is a precursor to tanning in those who actually do tan. The darker your natural skin tone, the less easily you burn— but you're still getting all that harmful radiation. Some people just burn and never tan, especially fair, red-headed, freckled, and blue-eyed types.

"Sunlight is the most devastating factor in hastening aging skin," according to Dr. Tom Sternberg, UCLA dermatologist. "For sunlight affects all the layers, including the top subcutaneous layer, in producing sagging and wrinkling. It is cumulative, permanent, and progressive." As much as 80 percent of the visible signs of aging are directly due to sun exposure.

If you're going to jog or walk as your form of daily exercise, do it in the early morning or late afternoon, or after sunset if possible. And you can still burn on cloudy days, so cover up.

### Watch Out for UVA Waves

Sun rays are comprised of wavelengths A, B, or C. Ultraviolet-light A waves are responsible only for short-term tanning during your first twenty-four hours in the sun, but penetrate deeply into the dermis and can cause long-term damage. This is why, when you hit the beach for the first time each season, you get such a dramatic color change right away. Visiting a tanning studio in order to prepare for your summer may protect you from burning because you'll have a base to start from. But you're still getting those longer, low-energy UVA waves at the tanning studio! Doctors used to think these waves weren't as dangerous as UVBs, however recently, it's been discovered that they can be just as harmful.

## UVB Waves and How They Affect Your Skin

The UVB waves are shorter, higher energy rays that do cause longer-term tanning and sunburn. They do so by stimulating *melanocytes* to make more melanin in the skin, which in turn makes it darken. In addition to affecting the superficial layers of the skin (the stratum granulosum), they deliver ultraviolet rays to the stratum corneum, the top layer of the skin. These UVB waves are strongest between 10:00 A.M. and 3:00 P.M.

Studies have shown that UVB rays (most plentiful in the summertime) affect both animals and humans by inhibiting the immune system. Researchers at the M.D. Anderson Cancer Center in Houston report that even chemical sunscreens can't prevent this effect—so all the more reason to avoid sunburn.

The shortest wavelength rays, UVC, are absorbed by the ozone layer in the earth's upper atmosphere. However, because of the depletion of the ozone layer, we may not be as protected from UVCs as we think, so it's vital that we protect ourselves.

## How Sunscreens Work

Sunscreens fall into three categories: absorbers, reflectors, and a combination of the two.

*Absorbers* have *para-aminobenzoic acid* (PABA) or related compounds as an essential ingredient. These must be absorbed into the skin to be effective. The PABA then absorbs UVBs. Another ingredient, *anthranilates*, are moderately effective against both UVAs and UVBs. State-of-the-art sunscreens contain *Parsol*, generically known as *arobenzone*, which is the best UVA blocker now available—much better in the UVA range than any of the previously developed chemicals in sunscreens.

*Reflectors*, or physical sunscreens, scatter or reflect ultraviolet rays. These chemicals are made up of *red petrolatum* or *titanium dioxide*, *zinc oxide*, or *talc*. Lifeguards seem to prefer reflectors, because they can see and feel their coverage and need not reapply as often as the lotion and cream absorbers that work their way into the skin.

## What Is SPF?

The *sun-protection factor* (SPF) is an index of degrees of protection in sunscreens against exposure to UVB rays, and they're graded from 2 to 50. A minimum SPF of 15 should be used by everyone, and children who have more delicate skin need somewhat more.

The SPF is arrived at by dividing the amount of time you can safely stay in the sun *with* a sunscreen by the amount of time you can safely stay in the sun *without* a suncreen. If you normally burn after fifteen minutes of intense sun, a sunscreen with an SPF of 10 will allow you to remain outside for 150 minutes without burning.

But wearing a higher SPF is no reason to decide it's okay to nap all afternoon under those blistering rays. The reason is that all tans indicate that you have some degree of radiation injury. Think of the sunscreen as helping to protect you from solar injury; the rest you have to do with your own good common sense.

Most dermatologists believe an SPF of higher than 20 doesn't provide any significant increase in protection. But since sunscreens are easily rubbed off by objects or clothing and melt away with perspiration, using higher SPFs is a form of insurance. Although some sunscreens are waterproof and are quite effective when tested after twenty minutes of swimming, no sunscreen is *completely* waterproof.

## Five Sunscreen Essentials

You should apply your sunscreen a half-hour prior to exposure, unless you're using a physical sunscreen such as zinc oxide, in which case you can put it on just before you go outside. Don't be stingy with any sunscreen product—the SPFs are based on liberal application. Better to be safe and sloppy than sorry and scarred. Also, if you're swimming or perspiring, reapply more frequently. Be especially vigilant if:

1. You're spending a lot of time in or on the water (swimming, boating, water skiing)

2. You're at the beach near the Equator.

3. You're at a high altitude. When you're in the mountains, there's less atmosphere to absorb the sun's rays.

4. It's summertime, between 10 A.M. and 3 P.M.

5. There's enough snow on the ground to reflect the sun.

## BUYING THE MOST EFFECTIVE SUNSCREEN

There are as many as forty pathological skin conditions relating to sun exposure, ranging from skin eruptions and sunburn to skin cancer. But thankfully, we can avoid most of them if we're really committed to applying sunscreen.

Suncreen products continue to improve. A broad-spectrum product is always best, covering the A, B, and C forms of ultraviolet rays.

Products with a high SPF have both a higher number and a greater volume of screening chemicals. Sunscreens come in many forms these days: lotions, creams, gels, and liquids that have alcohol bases and aerosol sprays. Some are scented, some unscented, and you may want to stay odorless if you don't want to attract bugs. Sunscreens with an alcohol base are better for those with oily skin.

Currently, a new product called *Prozone*, which contains a 1 percent concentration of the natural skin pigment, melanin, is in the research stage. It promises to be a highly effective, broad-spectrum sunscreen. Melanin has a natural antiaging effect on the skin due to its antioxidant properties, and we'll undoubtedly see more of it in skincare products as time goes by.

## Protect Yourself While Swimming

No matter what your race, your skin shading, or color, you still need to protect your skin from the sun. If you love swimming, you're in the sun on a routine basis—but you're also in the water, which washes off sunscreen. So it's important to know the difference between water-resistant (good for forty minutes of swimming) and waterproof (good for eighty minutes). But no matter how good a sunscreen is, once it's wiped off, you've got to reapply.

## Sun-Protective Clothing

There's a whole new line of SPF clothing to help keep your skin below the neck looking ten years younger. A soft, lightweight fabric is made from a nylon-based fiber woven to provide an SPF of at least 30. For swimming, there's a slightly stretchy version of this fabric that can be made into bathing suits. One particular product is made of nylon covered with an inert, nontoxic chemical which is able to block out 99 percent of UVB and 93 percent of UVA rays. Continued washings do not reduce the sunscreen effect. The FDA has begun to approve these garments for commercial use, so expect to see them in your stores soon.

## Protecting Your Eyes

The eyes are not only the window to the soul, they are also made up of extremely fragile and delicate tissue. As we age, they become increasingly susceptible to the harmful rays of the sun, become more bloodshot from the rupture of small blood vessels and are also prone to cataract development as the years go by. And then there are the wrinkles *around* the eye caused by squinting.

If you're out in the sun a lot, whether driving or exercising, you should be wearing sunglasses that protect you from UVB waves. But how do you know which to choose?

In 1986, the American National Standards Institute categorized the effectiveness of sunglasses into three categories:

❑ *Cosmetic*—which block 70 percent of UVB and 60 percent of UVA

❑ *General purpose*—which block 95 percent UVB and 60 percent UVA

❑ *Special purpose*—which block 95 percent UVB and 98.5 percent UVA

You can order glasses that effectively block *all* UVA and UVB waves from several companies around the country:

Eye Communications, (800) 247–5731

Noir Medical, (800) 521–9746

JS & A Blublocker Glasses, (800) 323–6400.

You can go into any eyeglass and lens store and get a long explanation as to why one type is preferred over another, but the sales help are generally trained to point you in the most expensive direction; in other words, you're usually paying more for a fancy frame. When you do select glasses, keep in mind that wraparound shades will keep the sun's rays from sneaking in at the corners.

## KEEPING YOUR SKIN CLEAN AND YOUNG

One way of looking ten years younger is to speed up the transit time of your cells, so that new, younger-looking cells will appear on the surface. You can do this with a washcloth and the proper cleansing agent. Using a scrub or cleansing grains will induce more rapid desquamation by taking off the old, dead cells on the top, the "horny" layer of the skin. In many individuals, it will accelerate the transit time as well, resulting in newer cells at the top layer. Not only will you look fresh and youthful, the exfoliation encourages and stimulates the formation of new skin cell generation from the basal layer.

What kind of cleanser should you scrub with? You can go the natural route and use a handful of cornmeal or oatmeal from your kitchen mixed with a little water, or you can go the commercial route and purchase products called cleansing grains, scrub cleansers, sloughing cleansers or washing grains. These usually consist of abrasive particles—natural ones such as apricot seeds, almonds or oatmeal, or synthetic ingredients such as silica or zirconium oxide—suspended in a cleansing cream. Scrubs for dry skin may include moisturizers or oils. And there are also scrubs for oily skin.

Take care not to overdo it, though. If you combine a scrub with a loofah or harsh washcloth, you may go too far too fast and end up with skin irritations. You must be extra careful of the delicate tissue around your eyes when you're scrubbing, since that particular area needs very gentle care.

If you have oily skin, scrub once a day. If you have dry skin, do it no more than every other day. If you have extremely dry skin, then this cleansing approach may not be appropriate for you, and you can simply use an astringent to keep your face clean and shining. Regardless of skin type, it's a good idea to follow up with a moisturizer after cleansing.

### Getting Rid of Wrinkles

If you have the time and money, you can choose from a number of options to bring about some radical changes in your face. Think long and hard before you do this, however. Your face is a map of your personality, and a few wrinkles are marks of character you can be proud of. Also, people who go through facial surgery sometimes feel terribly disoriented at first, as though they have lost their identity and find it unsettling to look at themselves in the mirror.

But each of us is different, and for some, a desire for real change is not just vanity, it's a matter of self-esteem. If you're in your forties or fifties, and you have been abusing your face for decades, you may have more wrinkles than you deserve. In that case, you might think about consulting a dermatologist or plastic surgeon about chemical peels or dermabrasion.

DERMABRASION. This process is a more intense version of the scrub. Typically, a dermatologist or plastic surgeon uses an instrument like a dental burr to abrade the surface of the skin. This is done as an office procedure under local anesthesia. This procedure can improve heavily aged skin and is also helpful in the treatment of acne rosacea.

The dermabrasion procedure goes beneath the horny layer down to the middle layers. As a result, a crust forms on the treated area which comes off after about a week. The area remains red and extremely sensitive for the next two to four weeks. This process shortens the transit time of cell generation through to the outer layers, resulting in younger, plumper cells at the surface. Dermabrasion is a very delicate procedure and must be done by a professional with a great deal of experience, since a bad job can cause permanent scarring. When you interview your doctor, ask if you can speak to other patients who've had success with dermabrasion.

CHEMICAL PEEL. Chemical peel, also called superficial chemosurgery or skin peeling, is performed by applying an acid to the skin. This causes the superficial layer to peel away, revealing a smoother, more youthful layer. At one time, carbolic acid or phenol was used, but this substance proved too toxic. These days, *sulfur* and *salicylic acid lotions* are used as well as the popular *benzoyl peroxide* and the controversial *tretinoin* (Retin-A).

RETIN-A. Retin-A had originally been used as a treatment for acne. Then, about ten years ago, a dermatologist at the University of Pennsylvania discovered that Retin-A not only accelerated transit time, but also stimulated blood vessel growth in the skin and boosted production of collagen and elastin, both of which decrease with the process of aging. The result is smoother skin with fewer wrinkles and lighter age spots.

Tretinoin is the active ingredient in both Retin-A and its oilier version, called *Renova*. It is a vitamin-A compound that will lessen fine lines (though not deep character lines), lighten brown spots and restore and revitalize skin that has been broken down by too much sun exposure. One new, exciting finding about tretinoin is that it actually fights cancer. In 1993, researchers at the University of Pennsylvania applied Retin-A to one side of the backs of patients with irregular moles that often turn cancerous. After six months, the treated side showed smaller moles which were no longer precancerous, while the moles on the other side remained unchanged.

Retin-A does have its drawbacks. It can cause extreme skin sensitivity. For the first few months of using the product, you must avoid irritating your skin with extremely hot or cold water, harsh washcloths, soaps or lotions, or skin products containing alcohol. You must avoid the sun as much as possible and always use a sunscreen outdoors. If you don't, you invite a bad burn and may actually accelerate the aging process and *increase* your risk of skin cancer.

Use of Retin-A is a lifelong commitment, since your skin will slowly revert to its normal state if you stop using it. But those who are loyal to Retin-A see a real improvement in their appearance, and it's the only product currently on the market that will really transform your skin.

## KEEPING YOUR SKIN SMOOTH AND CLEAR

There are other products, however, that will make somewhat of a difference in your skin texture and appearance. You may wish to consider *alpha hydroxy acids* (AHA); *bleaches*; and *collagen, fibrin,* or *fat* injections.

*Alpha Hydroxy Acids* (AHA). These come in the form of creams and lotions that are applied to the skin twice a day. They're primarily moisturizers, but they do speed up exfoliation as well and may smooth out the fine wrinkles and roughness. Sold by prescription as *Lac-Hydrin* or over the counter in weaker forms (Alpha Hydrox, Lac-

Hydrin Five, Anew), AHA falls somewhere between Retin-A and ordinary moisturizers in effectiveness.

The smallest of the AHA molecules penetrate easily and deeply into the skin. Alpha hydroxy acids may actually produce more collagen, a structural component of the skin, and act as an antioxidant to limit or prevent further sun damage.

Depending on the amount of AHA in the product you use, you may sense a tingling or sensitivity when you begin treatment. If you develop a rash, discontinue use of the product and try a milder version after the irritation has cleared up.

B*leaches.* Bleaches, such as *hydroquinone cream*, can be applied to discolored areas about twice a day. Minor discolorations will remain lightened for a few months after treatment ends. Not as effective as AHA and slightly more expensive, bleaches are available both in prescription form and half-strength in over-the-counter products. As with AHA, these may result in slight, temporary rashes in some individuals.

*Injections.* Injections of collagen (from cow hide), fibrin (gelatin made from pig tissue mixed with the patient's blood) or the patient's own fat (from the abdomen or thigh) can smooth fine wrinkles and other minor pits and grooves in the skin. Effects can last from a few months to two years. There have been several reports of skin damage and adhesions (scar tissue) under the skin from these injections, so investigate the procedure well before you choose it.

## Don't Buy the Package, Learn About the Product

We are all eager for miracles, but in fact, they rarely happen. Unfortunately, our society puts so much of a premium on youth and beauty that many of us are seduced into disregarding our own natural looks and trying to achieve an ideal image that's impossible, no matter how hard we try.

Women have been persecuted for decades by advertisers, who hold out the carrot at the end of the stick. If you use enough of this and enough of that, you just might look a blushing fifteen again. But real beauty doesn't come in a jar, and we should have a better perspective on where it does lie when we walk into a store looking for a product that will enhance our appearance.

No cosmetic product does anything other than make the skin moist and make it look smoother while it is on the skin. Cosmetic advertisements boast that certain ingredients have antiaging properties; however, except for AHA, which has an exfoliating ability and the sunscreen component of many cosmetics which protect you from photoaging, there is *no product* in the cosmetic department of a department store or beauty aisle of your drugstore that will actually make your skin younger.

I have to stress this because of the intense efforts advertisers go to in order to confuse customers. In the late 1980s, the cosmetic industry clashed with the Food and Drug Administration to resolve how far it could go in creating ads that claimed the antiaging properties of their products. The FDA finally decided, in their letter to the cosmetic companies, that "all of the examples that you use to allege an effect within the epidermis as the basis for a temporary effect on wrinkles, lines or fine lines are unacceptable."

What matters in the long run is not the brand of cosmetic you use, or the claims made by advertisers, but rather the day-to-day care and consideration you give your skin. The cardinal priority, as I mentioned earlier, is to keep your face clean, minimize the aging effect of the sun, and drink lots of water daily to keep your skin moist.

## Things You Never Knew About Soap

The most common cosmetic is soap, which is a mixture of sodium salts and various fatty acids of natural oils and fats, and comes in bars, granules, flakes, or liquids. Its basic function is to act as a catalyst for water and dirt to combine so that we can remove the resulting mixture from our skin.

In general, soaps don't add but subtract moisture from your skin, no matter what their ads say. Even if they contain moisturizers, these will be washed away along with the natural oils in your skin.

If you have thin, dry skin and a light complexion, you may find soap too drying. In that case, you should consider cleansing creams and lotions specially designed for sensitive skin.

Superfatted soaps have lanolin, oil, or cold cream added to them in order to replace some of the oils they wash away. But there is a question among dermatologists as to whether or not this works. It is unlikely that a soap can "choose" to wash away some oils while depositing others onto the skin and leaving them intact.

Soaps come in many forms, which makes for a great deal of confusion for the buyer. If a soap is advertised as an antimicrobial or antiacne product, it is regulated by the FDA as a cosmetic; otherwise, it's simply out there on the shelves. So it's hard to know a good soap from a bad one. It's also hard to know a soap from a detergent, for that matter. The difference is in the pH factor, or whether they are more acid or more alkaline.

The pH scale measures the degree of acidity (any value under 7) versus alkalinity (any value greater than 7). Under normal conditions, the skin is slightly acidic (pH = 4.5 to 6.5). Its *acid mantle*, as it's called, is a combination of dead skin cells, natural oils, and perspiration.

Soap is by nature *alkaline*, or *basic*—that is, it has a pH above 7. If a soap is too basic, it can have a somewhat irritating effect on dry skin. So if your skin type prefers non-alkaline cleansers, a detergent is the product you should choose. Detergents are reputed to be more drying to the skin than soaps, but some detergents have added emollients which make them even milder than the average soap, for example Dove, which is really a detergent and contains cold cream, as opposed to Ivory, which is an old-fashioned soap made by combining an alkali with fat and water.

### Moisturizing Products for Your Skin

After you've cleaned your skin with soap or detergent, it's important to use a moisturizer if you want to keep it looking ten years younger. Older skin tends to have less natural moisture, so you have to help it along.

### Causes of Dry Skin

As you get older, sweat glands and oil glands diminish in size and number, resulting in drier skin. Beyond that, some women have naturally drier skin than others. You can also dry out your skin prematurely by:

❐ using a very alkaline soap

❐ bathing too often (this washes away the protective oils of the skin)

❐ being exposed to dry air in winter, especially heated, blown air. The average humidity in a sealed, heated building is 10 percent or less; and anything less than 30 percent begins to have a drying effect on the skin. Aside from the protection of your moisturizer, you'll do your skin a favor if you place a pot of water on the radiator in every room, to restore a little humidity to the air.

Moisturizers are either emollients or humectants. You can use either to good effect if you want to keep your skin younger looking.

### EMOLLIENTS

1. *Petroleum jelly*—the best and cheapest moisturizer. Emollients are basically softening agents, specially developed to protect the skin by relieving dryness, promoting a softer, smoother skin. The emollient essentially works by forming a barrier through which water will not pass. By far, the most effective and least expensive emollient is petrolatum, known commercially as Vaseline. Tests at the University of Pennsylvania showed Vaseline to be the most effective moisturizer made, because it lasted for two weeks after the application! An additional benefit of Vaseline is that it is unscented and inert and very rarely causes allergic reactions. Beware of the variety advertised as having a "baby-fresh" scent, however, if you have sensitive skin that is prone to allergies.

2. *Lanolin*—the most natural emollient. The next best choice is lanolin, extracted from sheep wool. Lanolin is an important component of both expensive and inexpensive skin care products, but you can buy the ingredient by itself for maximum benefit. In addition to preventing the loss of moisture, it helps soften the skin, since it is very close in composition to your own natural oil secretions. The only drawback to this similarity is that lanolin, like natural oils, can make some women break out.

3. *Mineral oil*—the most common emollient. This is the least effective of the three as a moisturizer, yet it is the most common ingredient in skin care products.

### HUMECTANTS

Humectants, made of a chemical called *propylene glycol*, draw moisture from the air and then transfer it to the surface of the skin.

This doesn't work if the ambient air is very dry, however. In that case, the process reverses itself, drawing moisture from the skin. So humectants work best in a humid environment.

## CREAMS AND LOTIONS

All you really need to restore moisture to your skin is water. The trick is to keep the water on your skin. That's where oil comes in. A moisturizer is basically a mix of oil and water. If there's more oil and less water, you have a cream or ointment; more water and less oil, you have a lotion. Creams are more effective, but lotions are more popular because they blend into the skin more effectively.

If you can retain moisture and protect from the sun's harmful rays at the same time, you have all your bases covered. Since you're exposed to the sun traveling to and from work, outside when you're exercising, or when you're sitting near a window, you should be protected. Choose a moisturizer with sunscreen already in it, and you won't have to buy two different products.

The most important point about skincare is that you have to be adaptable, depending on what climate you're in. In cold weather, you need a richer cream to protect and nourish your skin. In warm weather, you need a lighter lotion and a sunscreen.

— SIDEBAR II —

## SOAP TRANQUILIZERS FOR YOUTHFUL SKIN
## AND A CALM MOOD

Scientists at the Memorial Sloan-Kettering's Psychiatry Service have experimented with the tranquilizing effects of a vanilla scent called *heliotropin* on patients undergoing magnetic resonance imaging (MRI). This test often induces claustrophobia because the patient is required to lie motionless inside a narrow tube for up to an hour. Results have indicated that those patients exposed to the fragrance were 63 percent less anxious than those who had no vanilla to smell. What if we could attach such an aroma to everyday soap? Could we become both clean *and* relaxed in one easy swipe? It's certainly worth investigating.

Scientists at Yale's Psychophysical Center have explored the use of lavender as a calming fragrance as well. You might want to try a lavender soap and see if it soothes your mind while it also soothes the skin on your face.

## Age-proof Your Skin with Vitamins

Now let's turn to the nutritional factors that affect your skin. You can protect your skin by ingesting vitamins, and sometimes by applying them directly to your face.

VITAMIN A AND RETINOIDS. Vitamin A, or its precursor, beta carotene, is found in yellow and green vegetables and is essential to the good health of your skin cells. Without it, skin becomes dry and scaly. Tretinoin, related to this vitamin, is the chief ingredient in Retin-A.

VITAMIN E. Vitamin E will also keep the skin in good condition, because of its antioxidant qualities. As we get older, we are more subject to the activity of free radicals, the wild chemical reactants which race through the body damaging tissue. These free radicals can be kept in check by antioxidants, and vitamin E is a crucial one for the skin. One useful property of this vitamin is that it can be applied directly to the skin and is therefore frequently found in skin creams and lotions.

Vitamin E works by direct application. But all other nutrients applied directly to the skin have no nutritional or healing effect— they are moisturizers, plain and simple. Avocado extracts and mink oil essences, for example, do not "feed" the skin. They only keep it moist.

VITAMIN C. Vitamin C provides many benefits to your skin, one of the primary ones being the maintenance of the structural integrity of your blood vessels. Since the skin is so sensitive to the blood supply directly underneath it, it stands to reason that C is vital to keep you looking younger.

THE B VITAMINS. In the absence of B vitamins, the skin may become red and begin to peel, dry cracks may appear at the corners of the mouth, and a scaly rash may develop on the face. Deficiency of $B_{12}$ can result in extreme pallor, and a deficiency of niacin ($B_3$) can cause pellagra. So to protect your skin, a B-complex vitamin should be part of your daily vitamin-mineral regimen.

Your skin, like the rest of your body, needs a balanced, healthy supply of nutrients, which can be found in the Ryback Food Plan (see Chapter Two). Good food is a great asset to your skin because your body can best absorb its vitamins and minerals directly rather than in supplemental form.

## Why Cigarettes and Alcohol Make You Look Old

Remember W.C. Fields' claim to fame? His red, bulbous nose was the facial signature of the chronic alcoholic. The condition he used to such advantage in his character is known as *rosacea*, and results from dilation of the blood vessels, often aggravated by excessive drinking. Although alcohol is only one factor that contributes to this condition, it's one we have direct control over if we so choose.

Excess alcohol may result in bloodshot eyes, which certainly ages the face. It also dehydrates the skin. Alcohol also disturbs the delicate balance of neurotransmitters that help us to fall and remain asleep. So when you wake up unrefreshed after too much alcohol, your skin really shows it.

Smoking not only keeps you from living ten years longer, it certainly prevents you from looking years younger. It's well known that smoking causes wrinkling and drying of the skin around the mouth by damaging the outer "barrier" layer of skin. In addition to prematurely wrinkling the facial skin, smoking also yellows the teeth and fingernails. Resins and tars from tobacco build up on the teeth, making plaque and tartar more difficult to remove.

Smoking allows carbon monoxide to replace the oxygen in the blood and otherwise narrows the blood vessels. This results in decreased oxygen flow to the growing skin cells, causing premature wrinkling in many smokers.

If you're having difficulty giving up cigarettes, see Chapter Ten for a full discussion of smoking cessation.

— SIDEBAR III —

### "ACHIEVING YOUNGER SKIN IN EVERY DECADE"

**Age 30:** As cell turnover begins to slow down, skin may start to appear somewhat duller. To look younger:

❐ avoid overexposure to the sun

❐ use broad-spectrum sunscreens

❐ consider superficial chemical peels

**Age 40:** Skin may begin to show discoloring or moles. It also thins out slightly. Crow's feet may develop around the eyes. To look younger:

❐ Talk with your dermatologist about Retin-A treatment

❐ Discuss the benefits of facial scrubs and dermabrasion

**Age 50:** Wrinkling becomes more prominent. To look younger:

❐ Use alpha hydroxy acids (AHA) in cream or lotion form to speed up the rate of exfoliation.

❐ Consider deep chemical peels.

**Age 60:** Fat pockets may form under eyes. Facial skin becomes slack and wrinkling increases. To look younger:

❐ Bleaches can be applied to discolored areas

❐ Injections of collagen, fibrin, or your own fat can reclaim your original, youthful contours.

❐ New technologies in plastic surgery may be worth considering.

**Age 70:** Your true character is now on display for the world, and you, to enjoy. You don't need to do a thing other than keep your skin clean and moisturized.

## Choosing the Best Makeup for a Youthful Appearance

Makeup cannot alter skin structure, although the advertising claims would like to leave you feeling that anything is possible. Cosmetics shade and enhance the different planes of your face, and that is all. They can bring out your good points and minimize your weak ones, and the best makeup job is the one that is so subtle, you can barely tell it's there.

So ignore the ads and the eager sales staff, and just consider the products you can purchase if you choose to. What works for you may not work for your best friend and vice versa. When deciding what to buy, follow these guidelines:

1. Never assume that the salesperson is right. Learn enough about your own skin coloring, texture, and tones to make an informed choice of your own.

2. If a salesperson is insistent about a new product, ask if you can return it if it doesn't work for you. Most reputable companies will stand by their product, or at least offer you an exchange if you don't like it.

3. Don't believe everything you see or hear in the ads. There are no "secret" or "miracle" ingredients. If something gives fantastic results, every cosmetics lab would analyze that product and duplicate it. So antiwrinkle creams are a fraud, as are eyelift creams. The only products that have a transforming physiological effect on the skin are sunscreens and Retin-A.

4. No cosmetics company has a monopoly on the best products. Each company has some good and some poor products. Choose according to specific product, not cosmetics line.

5. High cost does not equal effectiveness. Just compare the ingredients in high- and low-cost products and you'll be surprised to see how similar they are—except for the expensive packaging, of course.

6. Always buy the smallest amounts of a product at first to see how it works for you under different lighting, temperature, and humidity.

7. Always carry a small mirror with you when shopping for cosmetics. Before deciding to buy, walk outdoors and see how the sample you're trying looks in natural daylight. If you're trying to match a certain outfit, bring a piece of it with you to put up against the product on your skin.

## TEN BASIC PRODUCTS FOR YOUNGER LOOKING SKIN

Here are ten basic products that will help you look younger. Remember, when you're applying makeup, that older skin can act like a painter's canvas, picking up every dot of color and shading, and accentuating wrinkles and lines instead of concealing them. You may want to use *less* makeup and less vivid colors as you get older for a subtle, natural effect that will enhance rather than try to disguise your features.

## Foundations

Foundations come in liquids that are oil-based or water-based with extra emollients, a cream powder compact that goes on as a cream but dries to a powder finish, and cream in a stick or compact form. The most important thing is to get an exact match to your skin color.
For those of you with normal skin, try the cream-to-powder form. For a youthful texture, some liquid-to-powder products are also excellent. If you have oily skin, try an oil-free foundation of half-glycerin and half-talc. It may take you a while to learn to apply this makeup to best advantage, but when it works, it provides a light, natural look. If you have dry skin, try an oil-free product without alcohol. Avoid heavy or greasy products and colors that don't complement your skin tone.

## Concealers

To conceal the darker shading under your eyes, choose textures that are lighter than your own skin tone, or a neutral tone. Be sure to choose one that won't dry your skin because the skin around your eyes has fewer oil glands than the rest of your face. Put on the concealer first, blend it well, then put on the foundation. You can get some great, inexpensive concealers at your drug store.

## Finishing Powders

All pressed or loose powders are basically the same, so ignore ads that claim substantial differences. Avoid powders that contain oils if your skin is oily. The most youthful-looking powders are those with a natural tan or beige finish.

## Blushers

For those of you with normal to oily skin, try cream powder blush, and practice applying it to different planes of your face to get the most natural effect. You may want to pick a brown rather than a pink tone. What you don't want are bright rosy cheeks that look painted.

## Eyeshadow

For a natural look, flat, matte eyeshadows in gray or brown shades are the best. You can usually find a good eyeshadow in your drugstore.

## Lipsticks

Stick with matte colors. Any lipsticks containing clay or powder will tend to dry out your lips and result in a parched look. Lip glosses don't typically last long enough to keep your lips looking moist.

## Lip Pencils

It's nice to outline your lips and give them some definition, but don't spend more than $3 to $6 for this product, because they're all basically made of the same ingredients.

## Eye Pencils and Liners

There are many choices. The pencils give you more control, and the cakes with a brush give you a lot of variety, enabling you to create thin or thick lines. Avoid felt-tip eyeliners or liquids which produce a drawn-on effect that can make your eyes look smaller and older. Avoid pencils that smudge or smear because they're too greasy, or those that are too hard and crack off when you sharpen them. After applying, follow with eyeshadow to ensure a longer-lasting effect.

## Eyebrow Pencils

Choose a pencil with a drier texture for a youthful look. For a fuller, fresh look, you can add a brow gel with color which is brushed on through the brow or use it on its own, without the pencil.

## Mascara

Water-soluble products are the best, since they allow for easy removal. However, if you wear contact lenses and your eyes tear easily, you may want the waterproof variety. Experiment with different products until you find one that doesn't run, clump, smudge or flake.

You'll know when you're making the right choice about makeup when the end result makes you feel confident and upbeat, according to Hollywood cosmetics consultant, Rhonda Resnick. That's your best criterion for achieving younger-looking skin.

# AGE-PROOFING YOUR BODY SKIN

Your face, of course, is only a small portion of your body, and you can't neglect the rest of it if you're aiming for a look that's youthful all over. Now let's turn to the skin from the neck down and see what we can do to continue the antiaging process.

## What Is Cellulite?

What exactly constitutes the pitted, dimpled look of the skin on the thighs and buttocks of many women? Cellulite is a disruption of normal skin contouring caused by uneven layers of fat deposited under the surface. As you age, your skin loses its elasticity, especially if you don't keep your muscles firm through exercise and lean through proper nutrition. Genetics certainly plays a role, too, but fitness, diet, good posture, stress reduction and good circulation may also play a role.

The best medicine for cellulite is daily aerobic and isometric exercise. There are no special exercises aimed specifically at this problem. A full, consistent enjoyable routine of ongoing exercise—jogging, cycling, swimming, or brisk walking on the aerobic side and weight training on the isometric side—will do the trick over time. See Chapter Three for specific exercise advice.

Reducing cellulite is a very gradual process, and it's not always easy to find a solution that works for you. You cannot get rid of cellulite by using any special skin ointments. Anti-cellulite creams just don't work. Liposuction may be appropriate in some circumstances, but generally, it can be very disappointing. If the surgeon is unskilled or overeager, the result may be worse than the original problem. Contour irregularities or unnatural looking dents in the skin following liposuction are common. Once the surgery is complete, only dieting remains as an alternative solution, and the irregularities may persist even when you're thinner.

Speaking of losing weight, one thing that will not help cellulite is yo-yo dieting. That's the very self-destructive pattern of losing lots of weight and then regaining the same amount or more. When you throw the body's chemistry out of balance in this way, you may actually encourage cellulite to develop. The stretching and shrinking of your hips and thighs can weaken the elasticity of your skin, causing it to bump over the fat underneath.

There is no special anticellulite diet; however, my Antiaging Food Plan (see Chapter Two) is designed to help. The only additional diet aids reputed to assist in getting rid of cellulite are pineapple, papaya, mango, and kiwi. Supposedly these fruits contain enzymes which can increase the production of new collagen fibers in your skin.

If you want to work on your cellulite more rapidly and you're motivated to go beyond my Antiaging Food Plan, you might consider halving the portions I recommend on alternate days, and juggling the fruit and vegetable allotments. Eat only fruit on one assigned day and only vegetables the next. This program will give you a good balanced diet while significantly reducing your food intake. Cellulite isn't something to be ashamed of. Even if all your efforts to get rid of it are only making a slight difference, that's sufficient. Remember, this is your body, and you have a right to be proud of it. Eat less, stay fit and give looking ten years younger your best shot. You're here and you count—maybe for an extra ten years.

### Minimizing Varicose Veins

Varicose veins are abnormally enlarged blood vessels where blood has pooled, which makes them appear bluish and twisted. Blood flowing up the legs has to overcome gravity to get up to the heart, and it does so by moving through valves in the veins. These open as blood goes through and then shut tight to prevent backflow. However, if the valves weaken, blood can leak through and pool in the legs, causing the veins to dilate and bulge.

The valves are made up of tiny flaps of tissue that shut together when blood flows downward as the circulatory pressure tries to drive it upward. During the active phase of blood pressure (the *sys-*

*tole*), the blood is pushed upward and the valves open to allow the blood through. Then they close together during the *diastole* or resting period between heartbeats as the blood is pulled down by gravity.

When one valve in a vein fails, the one just below has to carry the extra strain. If that valve fails, then the valve below gets the burden, and so on, like a stack of dominos falling over. The good news is that this process of deterioration is gradual, so if you have the beginnings of a problem with varicose veins, don't panic. Your circulatory system is incredibly resilient and won't fall apart quickly or easily.

WHY VARICOSE VEINS?  One women in five will have varicose veins during her lifetime. Genetics is the strongest risk factor. But the next most prevalent problem is the occurrence of a *thrombosis*—a blood clot at the site of a valve—which can occur during pregnancy, major surgery, or during an accident.

A great number of women see varicose veins popping out when they are pregnant. The growing uterus (and the extra weight you're carrying) presses on the veins in the pelvis, resulting in an increase of pressure in the leg veins and ultimately, in the veins on the surface of the legs. *Vulval veins*, around the entrance to the vagina, may appear at the beginning of the second trimester. A big factor here is that higher progesterone levels during pregnancy relaxes the muscles in the legs, increasing your susceptibility to varicose veins— which, by the way, tend to improve after childbirth.

Other contributing factors to varicose veins include poor diet, lack of exercise, and standing on your feet all day in one position. Although taking oral contraceptives doesn't cause varicose veins, it may increase your risk of thrombosis, especially after age 35. You should discuss the advisability of taking the Pill or hormone replacement therapy with your physician if you have a problem with varicose veins or any other type of thrombosis.

Spider veins are small varicose veins that appear as bluish or reddish lines under the surface of the skin and commonly appear on the upper leg and lower thigh. They present no health problem whatsoever. However, if you are very unhappy with the look of them, they can be treated with *sclerotherapy* (see treatments that follow), by heat, or with electrolysis. These treatments are not always successful, however, often leaving a brown discoloration on the skin which may be more noticeable than the original spider veins. If you feel terribly self-conscious about these veins, you can always cover them with makeup.

ANTIAGING SOLUTIONS FOR YOUR VEINS. A slim body is the first defense against varicose veins, so I urge you to follow my Antiaging Weight Loss Program (see Chapter Two) in order to keep your weight under control. A daily exercise regimen is just as vital as your nutrition; you can use my SPEAR program (Chapter Three) to help you get started. In addition to your regular exercise routine, there are some special leg exercises you can do to help prevent varicose veins. All of these are performed lying down, and you can do them in bed, right after you awaken each morning. That way, you'll begin your day with your blood pumping and energy flowing.

1. Lie on your back and point your toes down away from you toward the foot of the bed. Then flex your toes and curl them upward toward your head as much as you can. Repeat 5 to 10 times.

2. In the same position, place your feet about a foot apart. Circle each foot inward and continue the circle back to your starting position. Be sure you touch all points along the circle. Make five circles inward, then reverse and make five circles outward.

3. On your back, tense each leg alternately, keeping your knees straight. Hold each leg up about two feet off the mattress and then lower it slowly. Repeat five times a day during the first month, ten times a day the second month, and twenty times a day from the third month on.

4. While still on your back, raise your legs and cycle them slowly ten times. After a month, double the number of repetitions, then double again after another month. This is the most important of the four exercises in terms of overall leg strength, flexibility, and cardiovascular challenge.

If you're forced to stand in one place on the job, try subtle exercises that you can perform without anyone noticing. Transfer your weight from foot to foot, stretch up on your toes slightly, then sink your weight as you bend your knees. Whenever you can, sit with your legs raised on a stool or ottoman or another chair. If you're home watching TV, lie on the floor and prop your legs up on a pillow or hassock. Better yet, ride your exercise bike or rowing machine as you watch your favorite show.

NONSURGICAL AND SURGICAL SOLUTIONS. Options for treatment include wearing elastic stockings, sclerotherapy (injections that cause the affected veins to die off), and surgical stripping of the veins.

Elastic stockings give the veins support and keep them from dilating abnormally. These stockings help to squeeze the blood out of the smaller veins near the skin and into the larger, stronger veins deeper inside.

Sclerotherapy involves a series of injections with a special solution that causes the walls of the vein to stick together, preventing blood from pooling there. The process forces the blood flow from the affected vein to those that are functioning effectively. There is no scarring with this procedure, which is why it's become so popular. This procedure is useful both for spider veins and for many varicose veins. In some stubborn cases, though, the doctor will tie off larger varicose veins under local anesthesia.

Your first session takes about an hour, and subsequent injections take only fifteen minutes. The number and size of your veins will determine how many treatments you will need.

After the injections, you'll wear elastic stockings for three to six weeks, and the leg will be firmly bound from the toes to the injection site. As the veins heal, they will gradually shrink, harden, and disappear. Walking and elevation seem to speed the healing process—it's a good idea to walk three miles a day and keep your legs raised in bed at night on pillows.

Surgery is the most drastic solution and is reserved for the most severe cases, most often for those who are obese and whose varicose veins extend up the thigh into the groin area. A surgeon will probably cut into the skin and strip out or tie off the affected saphenous vein from the groin to the knee. If there are other varicose veins below this point, they can usually be treated with sclerotherapy. This surgery is done on an outpatient basis and generally takes under an hour. You can go back to your regular activities within two days, as long as you're not engaging in heavy physical labor. For the next two weeks, you'll wear a compression bandage with foam padding cut to conform to the veins, held in place by several layers of elastic wrap.

These procedures may or may not hold up over time. About thirty percent of all individuals who undergo these procedures develop new varicosities within the next ten years. But if they do come back, you can always repeat the sclerotherapy process.

If you don't yet suffer from varicose veins, your best efforts at minimizing your chances of developing them are to eat right and exercise on a regular basis. The more you walk, the better your legs will look!

## Inexpensive Cosmetic Surgery for Your Eyes

Plastic surgery is not something to be entered into lightly (or inexpensively), but for those who are truly unhappy with their appearance, it may be a wise choice. An eyelift, for example, may provide a great psychological lift for a woman who feels her eyes tell the world she looks tired.

One alternative to conventional eye surgery is a new microliposuction technique. This relatively inexpensive procedure involves making a small incision at the site of a wrinkle in the corner of the eye and vacuuming out the undesirable accumulations of fatty tissue just under the eye. This results in a more youthful look without the expense of a traditional operation.

## Younger Looking Hands

Other than the face, the hands and nails are probably the most noticeable parts of our body. Of course, the need for sunscreen goes without saying—it's not just your face that needs protection. But sunscreen won't protect the hands from "liver spots" that may begin to develop in our thirties and become quite evident in our forties and fifties.

WHAT ARE LIVER SPOTS? These marks may be liver-colored, but they have nothing to do with the liver. They develop because of a genetic predisposition and exposure to the sun, which accelerates the process of discoloration.

You can generally hope to erase liver spots within six months of Retin-A treatments. Or you may opt for the process in which the spots are frozen with liquid nitrogen and then a bleaching agent is applied as the skin heals. Mild skin peels can also be used, but they are generally not as successful on the hands as they are on the face.

To take care of fine wrinkles on the hands, you can have them injected with collagen, which pumps up the creases. But this is a temporary solution and needs to be repeated from time to time in order to maintain the look. Because of the danger of adhesions (scar tissue) forming beneath the surface of the skin, most dermatologists don't often recommend this option.

You don't need to do a lot to your nails to keep them looking attractive. Good diet and hygiene are generally all you need. Pushing back the cuticles very gently and keeping the nails filed flat and round with an emery board will do the trick. In order to help nails maintain their natural strength and resilience to the stresses and strains of everyday life, it's advisable not to file them to a point. You can paint your nails with a hardener before polishing with clear or colored polish—or leave them natural.

How to Care for Your Cuticles. Cuticles can be pushed back when they grow onto the nail itself. It's best to do this right after your bath or shower when the skin is softest. If you get a lot of excess growth, you can clip the cuticles gently, but never all the way to the base or sides of the nail. Never cut or scrape into the nail border as this may result in pain and/or infection at the sensitive juncture. Never probe under the cuticle border with a sharp instrument. This very delicate area is where your nails are formed and develop.

What Not to Put on Your Nails. Many women go overboard and actually damage their nails with too many products. The glues used to apply false nails and acrylic processes tend to destroy the natural surface structure of the nail. Formaldehyde is a particularly unhealthy substance for nail surfaces. Stay away from acetone polish removers; they do a quick job on polish, but also dry out and damage the surface of the nail.

## AGE-PROOFING YOUR HAIR

For most of us, if we live long enough, we'll go gray. It's part of the inexorable aging process. Over time, we make less collagen which results in less color in the hair shaft. The hair is stripped of its original color, and even the texture changes over time, becoming coarser and less shiny.

## Do You Want to Color Your Hair?

Highlighting and semipermanent color are the best covers for early gray. It's a good idea to have these done professionally at a salon, where your hair can be evaluated and color matched to your original tone. If you decide to color your hair yourself, use a semipermanent treatment that sinks into the hair shaft and changes color by chemical reaction. Instead of leaving obvious signs of demarcation as time goes by, the color simply fades away, and the natural nuances of your original color will return. The effect usually lasts up to twenty shampoos or six weeks, whichever comes first. Highlighting treatments are also commercially available—by pulling only certain hairs through a plastic cap and tinting them, you achieve a lighter look overall, and a nice lift to your face reflected off the sunny highlights surrounding it.

## Maintaining Your Hair's Youthful Shine

As you mature into your forties, the volume of your hair tends to shrink, making the texture finer, limper, and more fragile. As you enter middle age, your scalp tends to become drier as your oil glands become less active. Choose shampoos and conditioners geared for dry hair, and take it easy with the hair dryer, curling iron, and hot rollers which will all dry out your hair. During the winter, hot-oil treatments may help as well.

— SIDEBAR IV —

### HOW TO HAVE YOUNGER-LOOKING HAIR

In the forties, hair tends to become thinner and more fragile and the scalp becomes drier. You can maintain your hair better if you:

- ❏ Keep your hair from becoming even drier from overexposure to the sun.
- ❏ Keep your hair healthy from within by sticking with the vitamin regimen recommended in Chapter Two.
- ❏ Consider changing your hairstyle to a shorter, bolder cut.

- ❏ If you want to color your hair, use henna and vegetable dyes as opposed to chemical permanent hair dyes. They're gentler to the hair shaft and more natural looking.
- ❏ Permanents tend to dry out the hair; you might want to try a body wave instead.
- ❏ Experiment with shampoos and conditioners until you find those that are right for you. Don't use the same products on your hair every day.
- ❏ Minimize use of blow dryers, curling irons, and hot rollers. Heat is an enemy to hair.
- ❏ Give yourself hot-oil treatments, particularly during cold weather when the hair follicles tend to dry out from overheated air.

## Are You Losing Your Hair?

Slight hair loss is to be expected as we get older. Older hair falls out or is pulled out during brushing, and new hair doesn't grow in as readily. This turnover process is normal and natural.

If you remember your pregnancy, your hair became suddenly lustrous and thick. The reason was the increased estrogen and progesterone in your system. Then, after childbirth, as your hormones returned to their normal level, your hair probably came out in handfuls—again, this is just nature's rebalancing process.

Women in midlife may find that, due to the declining levels of gonadal hormones, they aren't seeing as much regrowth of hair as they might like. Taking your vitamin and mineral supplements is important in addition to keeping up with a healthy nutrition program (see Chapter Two). Crash dieting can be devastating to your hair, as can certain medications.

Balding is typically a male problem, but about thirty million women in America also suffer from baldness, known as *androgenetic alopecia*. These women appear to have an abundance of male hormones, or androgens, and their hair-loss patterns are therefore more similar to those of a man.

Since women have less hair on their scalps than men, hair loss of 10 to 15 percent can be very noticeable. Unlike men, women experience hair loss diffusely over the entire scalp as opposed to one specific area.

Although a completely shaven head seems to be a fashion statement these days, most women are extremely self-conscious about balding. There are steps you can take to halt or slow the process, but you should have a full work-up by an endocrinologist before considering these treatments:

ELECTRICAL STIMULATION. The use of electricity is somewhat controversial, but the treatment is designed to "wake up" the quiescent follicles in your scalp as you sit under a hairdryer-like hood for twelve minutes while your scalp is bathed in a low-level electrical field. A dermatologist from the University of British Columbia found a two-thirds increase in hair counts in his research subjects from this treatment.

DRUGS. Hormone replacement therapy (see Chapter Five) may restore and replenish your hair, and may give it a youthful shine as well. This medication replaces your diminishing supply of estrogen and progesterone, the hormones that help to make your hair appear younger.

You may also want to consider taking *Rogaine* (minoxidil). About two-thirds of those who use it find that it successfully prevents further hair loss, and about one third find that it actually causes significant regrowth of hair after a six-month treatment. It's fairly expensive, though, costing upwards of $60 a month.

A somewhat new drug is *Proscar* (finasteride), first developed to treat prostate gland enlargement in men, but found to counteract baldness as well. Proscar works by preventing the formation of androgens which are involved in the demise of scalp follicles. Other baldness-fighting drugs currently being researched are *Tricomin*, which works by incorporating protein into the hair shaft, and the enzyme *aromatase*, which works by encouraging follicular activity in the scalp.

## AGE-PROOFING YOUR TEETH

Your teeth, like your bones, need more care and attention as you get older. The alignment in your jaw shifts subtly over time. In your forties, your teeth may begin to move around slightly, causing crookedness, crowding, or gaps. By now, some of the fillings you've had since you were a teenager may begin to wear around the edges, and your gums may begin to recede. By the time you're in your fifties, your teeth are more brittle and susceptible to breakage if you bite down on a hard object. Your teeth may also begin to discolor, both because of the accumulated effect of food stains or tobacco, and because of the thinning of tooth enamel which reveals the yellow dentin under the enamel.

## How to Keep Your Gums from Receding

In order to keep your teeth looking ten years younger, visit your dentist twice a year for a cleaning and general inspection. Keeping your teeth free of tartar or plaque will help keep your gums strong and supple so that they won't recede. Another must, regardless of age, is proper brushing and flossing. Check with your dentist for the proper technique. If you're too rough, or use a back-and-forth instead of a circular brushing pattern, you may be fostering a  prematurely receding gum line. Another good preventive tip is to use a rubber-tipped toothbrush and massage your gums with it daily.

## Contouring and Veneers

There are many available options for making your mouth look younger and healthier. You may want to consider contouring or shaping your teeth. It may just be a matter of polishing the edges of a couple of teeth to make them appear more attractive.

If your teeth are discoloring, you can ask your dentist about bleaching, bonding, or using porcelain veneers. These processes can really work wonders to give your smile a new lift. Even the gaps between teeth can sometimes be improved by judicious use of veneers. And they may obviate the need for tooth replacement if you should happen to chip one.

— SIDEBAR V —

### Maintaining Younger Teeth

**Age 30:** Teeth may begin to discolor.
- tooth enamel thins

**Age 40:** Teeth may move slightly, causing crookedness or gaps.
- gums may begin to recede
- old fillings may deteriorate

**Age 50:** Teeth become more brittle and susceptible to breaking.

**Preventive Care:**

    1. Proper brushing and flossing.

    2. Twice-a-year visits to your dentist for inspection and cleaning.

    3. Consider bleaching, bonding, or porcelain veneers.

    4. Consider contouring or reshaping teeth that may have shifted.

## PUTTING IT ALL TOGETHER

Your skin, hair, and teeth are the most visible parts of you, and you owe it to yourself to keep them in good condition. Having taken responsibility for your appearance, you'll find it easier to start thinking about the internal processes that support the external structure. Remember, the way you look and feel doesn't depend solely on cosmetics, hair coloring, or a bright, fresh smile. Rather, a younger look also comes from within; from your attitude about your body and mind as well as your dedication to good nutrition and exercise.

When you have it all together, you will look ten years younger, and you'll know what to do to stay that way as you age.

# KEEPING
## YOUR HEART STRONG AND YOUNG

## CHAPTER 9

$H$ave you ever experienced a stabbing or squeezing pain in the center of your chest? And did you just decide that it was heartburn or gas, and choose to dismiss it? It's possible that what you felt was angina, which is one of the first signs of heart disease—a sign that you shouldn't ignore.

## WOMEN AND HEART DISEASE

Heart disease is the number one killer of American women. About a quarter of a million women each year succumb to the ravages of this illness. Six times as many women die from heart attacks as die from breast cancer every year in the United States; this is also a greater number than those who will die of all forms of cancer in women combined.

The great tragedy is that no one takes this information to heart. (Excuse the pun.) There are countless women in this country with serious heart disease who never tell anyone about those twinges. One-third of all heart attacks among women never get reported to physicians. There are two reasons for this: either the attacks are silent—without symptoms—and the women themselves don't know that they've had an attack; or, although the attacks are excruciatingly painful, the women deny that anything serious has happened. Women, who tend to handle pain better than men, often don't complain when they should. They don't realize that they are doing even more damage to their heart by not getting treatment.

Although fewer women than men experience a heart attack as their first symptom of coronary disease, those who do are twice as likely as men to die after their first heart attack and two times more likely than men to have a second attack or a stroke. Their chances of dying after coronary bypass surgery are twice that of men and they have lower success rates from treatments such as balloon angioplasty.

Women are also not as readily referred to a major cardiac center after a heart attack. Studies have shown that it usually takes twice as much time for women to be transferred to a specialized facility for further evaluation and treatment.

The medical establishment is only now becoming more enlightened to the facts about women's heart disease. There are still doctors who attribute women's cardiac complaints to indigestion, fatigue, menopause, or depression. Studies in Portland, Oregon and Boston, Massachusetts show that doctors are more than twice as likely to order diagnostic exams such as a treadmill test or cardiac catheterization for men as they are for women. Few women have an exercise test as part of an executive physical, though it's a routine procedure for men over 40.

Most of the clinical trials for heart medications have included men only, so it's difficult to judge whether many FDA-approved drugs and their dosages will be as effective in the female body.

From 1977 to 1993, the FDA banned women from early drug trials. Women were specifically excluded because it was thought that they might be in the earliest stages of pregnancy when they signed up for the trials, and the developing fetus might be damaged by the unknown effects of certain drugs. Although this ban has been lifted, there are still fewer clinical trials performed on women than men.

In the past, half of all the drug-safety experiments excluded women, and even those that did include them were judged incorrectly. Since women have more fat content in their bodies, a drug that's absorbed and held in fat lingers longer. Logically, this means that a woman can be given a smaller dosage to get the same effect that a man would get. But since the data on drug testing was often not separated, no indication was given that various drugs and their side-effects affected women differently than men. As a result, these medications might be ineffective or even damaging to the women taking them.

Many clinical trials conducted on men have shown that a daily aspirin is effective for men as a preventive measure to thin the blood and prevent clots. Will it work for women as well as it does in men? One large study on a group of nurses indicates that the answer is yes, but we won't know definitively until more women-only clinical trials take place.

We still think of heart disease as a man's illness, probably because men tend to have massive attacks which kill them quickly and dramatically. The female picture of an attack is quite different. It may do incredible damage to the heart without killing, yet leave the woman in a completely debilitated state. Women live typically eight to ten years longer than men, which means they face years of potential pain and disability.

The prevalence of heart disease has been decreasing for men since the 1950s while it has steadily increased for women. The truth of the matter is that after age 65, when their estrogen production is diminished and women lose the protection that this hormone affords the heart, they are just as vulnerable as their male counterparts.

So part of the discrepancy in our thinking about this disease has to do with the fact that it takes women twenty years longer than men to develop heart disease, and they may have other medical problems such as diabetes or osteoporosis. If they haven't been vigilant about preventive health care for that long, they are not just older, but sicker, when they start feeling the first twinges of angina.

Fortunately, there are new prospects for research and therapy. The Women's Health Initiative, sponsored by the National Institutes of Health, is a $625 million, ten-year research project that is currently addressing the health concerns of all older women. And as research forges ahead to discover new ways to keep the female heart young and healthy, we will hopefully see a decline in the rates of disease.

However, we can't wait around for science. We must take the first preventive steps ourselves. If you know what your risk factors for heart disease are, you can do everything in your power to lower or eliminate them.

## Female Risk Factors for Heart Disease

Why might you be susceptible to heart disease? The major risk factors are:

- ❑ Sex
- ❑ Age
- ❑ Family history
- ❑ Race
- ❑ Cholesterol levels
- ❑ Triglyceride levels
- ❑ Stress
- ❑ Cigarette smoking
- ❑ Smoking and birth control pills
- ❑ High blood pressure
- ❑ Obesity
- ❑ Diabetes

These factors all clearly interrelate, and the more you have, the more like you are to succumb to heart disease. Some factors you can change; others you can't. Let's talk about what steps you can take to make your heart profile as healthy as possible.

1. *Sex.* It's true that men succumb to heart attacks about ten to fifteen years earlier than women, but that doesn't mean that female gender lowers your risk forever—it simply delays it. Your female hormones also play a big part in your heart profile, because estrogen helps to keep your lipid profile in good balance. The decline of estrogen after menopause is a significant problem for some women. If you have a family history of heart disease, you may want to discuss estrogen replacement with your physician.

2. *Age.* By age 65, your risk of heart disease rises to equal that of a man. The older you are, the more likely you are to have other factors on this list such as high blood pressure, obesity, as well as other diseases, that would make you more susceptible to heart failure.

3. *Family history.* If you have any immediate family members who had heart disease under the age of 55, you are at greater risk yourself.

4. *Race.* African-American, Hispanic, and some Native American women have more risk factors than Caucasian women, and are therefore at higher risk.

You may not be able to change any of the above factors, but you can do a lot to counteract the following:

5. *Cholesterol levels.* You need to keep your "good" and "bad" cholesterol in the right proportion—that is, you want an HDL (high-density lipoprotein) level of more than 45 and an LDL (low-density lipoprotein) level below 130. The total should be less than 200.

6. *Triglyceride levels.* This particular lipid is more significant in women and can be an independent stress factor for them. Women are likely to have high triglycerides if they are overweight, have high blood pressure or thyroid dysfunction or if they abuse alcohol. Your triglycerides should be below 200.

7. *Stress.* If you are always on the edge of your chair, keyed up and anxious, you can create stress hormones that can cause arrhythmic heartbeats and raise blood pressure. The increase in pressure may have adverse effects on the blood vessel walls and allow plaque to be deposited there.

8. *Smoking.* If you're a smoker, you have virtually selected a shorter life span, but if you stop, you can easily add ten years to your life, and look and feel younger as well. Smoking not only affects your heart and lungs, but all your organs and your general fitness level.

9. *Smoking and birth control pills.* Estrogen and progesterone contained in the Pill enhance the body's ability to form blood clots. If you add cigarettes to this mixture, you contribute to possible heart attack, stroke, or pulmonary embolism.

10. *High blood pressure.* This condition is quite common in our culture. The picture of the "Type A" individual—a fast-track, aggressive, impatient, hot-tempered person who is ahead of the game in everything but health—has hypertension written all over it. But you don't have to fit this picture to be at high risk. Most people with hypertension feel great, until they have a heart attack or stroke. Blood pressure increases with age, so even if you are within normal range now, you may expect it to rise as you get older. But you can manage blood pressure effectively with vitamin and mineral supplementation in

addition to diet and exercise. The upper range of normal blood pressure is 140 (systolic pressure) over 90 (diastolic pressure). Anything higher is considered hypertensive.

11. *Obesity.*You shouldn't be more than twenty percent over your ideal weight range. Too much weight is a stress on all the body's organs; the heart in particular has to pump harder when you are lugging around those many extra pounds.

12. *Diabetes.* Diabetes mellitus lowers the body's ability to balance blood sugar levels and it can also lower HDL cholesterol. Some women with diabetes also have high blood pressure. This is not always a controllable risk factor, but it can be managed.

There are other factors that come into play when we're looking at the total heart picture. For example, your exercise level is crucial to management of heart disease. If you're really active, you bump up your HDL level even if you haven't changed your diet very significantly. Exercise also enhances the elasticity of your blood vessels so that the blood can flow better.

Alcohol consumption is a controversial risk factor—a small amount appears to increase HDLs; however, large amounts of alcohol can contribute to the development of heart disease.

An interesting risk factor is social isolation. Because the mind does affect the body, it is a proven fact that if our heart is lonely or sad, it can in fact get sick. Older women in our society are very often alone. Their spouses die on average six years before them, and their grown families may have moved far away. Women with no support system are less likely to get well when they're ill. As well, getting started in the morning is more difficult if they have no one counting on them.

Finally, you are better protected from heart disease if you are affluent and educated. As is true with many other conditions, you have to know a little about them to recognize risks and get symptoms treated when they appear. Poor, uneducated women also have trouble affording appropriate health care.

## The Estrogen Connection

Estrogen, that amazing hormone, is in great part responsible for women's healthy hearts prior to menopause:

❏ Estrogen helps in the production, maintenance and breakdown of HDL cholesterol and LDL cholesterol and keeps them in proper balance.

❏ Estrogen has a direct effect on the coronary arteries that supply the heart with blood. It keeps plaque formation low by blocking the LDLs from attaching to artery walls.

❏ Estrogen helps to keep the tone of blood vessel walls, and ensures their elasticity.

After menopause, however, when women's supply of estrogen drops to within 20 percent of their previous levels, they lose the beneficial effects mentioned above. And for those women who have a family history of heart disease, it may be a good idea to consider replacement hormones. Several studies have shown that women who take estrogen after menopause reduce their risk of heart disease by 30 to 50 percent.

It should be pointed out that it is the estrogen, not the progesterone, that is protective of your heart, and many experts feel the best candidate for hormones is the woman who has had a hysterectomy and therefore doesn't have to take progestin to protect the lining of her uterus. But other studies claim benefits for both hormones. (The elevated risk of breast cancer, though, is still something you have to take into consideration when you're thinking about replacement hormones.) See Chapter 5 for a full discussion of HRT and ERT.

Estrogen can be found naturally in several plant sources commonly used in Japanese cooking, so it's wise to protect your heart by increasing your consumption of miso, tofu and tempeh (soy products), as well as Siberian ginseng which may also act as a calming agent if you're under much stress.

## Pregnancy and Your Heart

If you are still in your reproductive years, and producing lots of estrogen, you may think you are totally protected from heart disease. This isn't so. Coronary artery problems have been shown to start at preschool age. In autopsies done on children as young as three (who had died of other causes), it was found that there were the beginnings of plaque on the arteries.

Young women are also prone to other heart ailments, such as arrhythmias and valve problems. These difficulties can be exaccerbated during pregnancy, when the body is working overtime to care not just for itself but for the growing baby within.

If you are considering getting pregnant, and you have been diagnosed with any heart problem, it's important to have an EKG (electrocardiogram) to establish a baseline for your heart. This way, you can be rechecked every subsequent trimester. Your obstetrician may want to refer you to a cardiologist for this specialized care.

During normal pregnancy, even a healthy heart has extra work to do as it supplies blood and nutrients to the growing fetus. The extra weight and pressure on your internal organs is also difficult for the heart and circulation. A variety of problems, from varicose veins to extra fluid in your legs (*edema*), may result from the burden on your heart. By your fifth month, your blood supply can increase by 50 percent, and the heartbeat elevates by the third trimester. The greatest challenge to the heart is the labor and delivery, when the heart must pump five times as hard as it normally does. (Labor is purported to be the hardest physical work you'll ever do in your life.)

If you're prone to high blood pressure, you'll really need to monitor it during your pregnancy. A case of *pregnancy-induced hypertension* (PIH) can lead to a dangerous condition called *toxemia* or *preeclampsia* in one out of four cases. If untreated, this can lead to maternal *eclampsia*, a condition that may involve convulsions, coma, and even death.

Those at greatest risk for PIH are African-American, first-time mothers under 35 with a history of high blood pressure and heart problems, diabetes, or obesity. You may suspect that your blood pressure is rising rapidly if you are experiencing a lot of edema and your shoes or gloves suddenly don't fit. Other symptoms are blurred vision, headaches that won't go away, and dizziness or pain in the upper abdomen. A special diagnostic urine test will identify you as a high-risk candidate, and if you're found to be in danger of PIH, you may be told to take a daily aspirin and get a lot of bed rest. Some women with the condition may have to be confined to bed for the last few weeks of their pregnancy.

A more typical circulatory problem during pregnancy is anemia. The normal level of hemoglobin (red blood cells) in the blood is about 12 grams, but it can dip to half that in anemic women. One of the biggest needs a pregnant woman has is for folic acid, which helps to produce red blood cells. The red cells are essential to the healthy development of your baby, since they carry oxygen to all the organs via the placenta. If you don't have enough red blood cells to do the job, your heart has to pump more blood to supply your fetus, and this can leave you feeling exhausted. Be sure you get 800 mg. of folic acid daily if you're pregnant to avoid anemia.

Occasionally, pregnant women develop heart irregularities. If you feel that you are having palpitations, rapid heartbeat, extra beats, or skipping a beat, be sure to tell your doctor. These symptoms are usually nothing to worry about and may actually be brought on by anxiety about the impending birth. Once you're aware of the reason for your symptoms, they may vanish without needing any treatment whatsoever.

## What Might Go Wrong with Your Heart?

1. *Coronary Artery Disease. Arteriosclerosis* (or atherosclerosis), occurs when fatty deposits or plaques develop on the inside walls of the coronary arteries. The passageway for blood is therefore narrowed, and the walls themselves harden. As they lose their elasticity over time, it gets harder for oxygenated blood to flow through them, and the blood supply to other organs may then get cut off. If a piece of plaque breaks off, it can cause an *occlusion*, or blood clot. The clot can block the artery completely. When the blood supply to a part of the heart muscle is cut off, it causes a *myocardial infarction* (heart attack).

You don't have to have a heart attack to have symptoms of cardiovascular distress. When there's sufficient blockage in an artery, or in several arteries, the heart can no longer receive enough oxygen and the pain of *angina*, a spasm from a temporary narrowing of the artery, results. Angina is described, alternately, as a crushing or squeezing pain which often radiates up to the jaw or down the left arm. How do you know that the angina you're experiencing isn't a heart attack? Classic angina goes away when you sit down and rest; but if you're having a myocardial infarction, no change of position or activity level will take the edge off the pain.

2. *Hypertension.* Hypertension is a more significant risk factor for women than men. Women with high blood pressure are nearly four times more likely to have heart disease than those with normal pressure, as opposed to men, who are three times more likely.

When this condition occurs, the heart has to work harder during each contraction. High blood pressure creates *shear stresses* on the artery walls, which can rupture existing plaques and start the clotting system—which may in turn lead to a heart attack.

Blood pressure is regulated by a fluid and nerve axis along the kidneys, brain and blood vessels. If something disturbs this axis, blood pressure changes. There's a lot of force pushing against the arterial walls each time the heart beats and, over time, this can severely damage them. A person with systemic hypertension may have thickened and enlarged heart walls, and this can eventually lead to heart problems. The kidneys and eyes can also be affected by hypertension—kidney failure and a particular form of blindness called *serous chorionic retinopathy* can result.

3. *Arrhythmias.* The normal beat of the heart is maintained by the electrical impulses that start in the *sinus node* and move to the various other locations in the heart. But if this rhythmic pattern is disturbed for any reason, there may be a temporary pause in a heartbeat, or perhaps an extra, additional beat. If arrthymias go on over a protracted time period, the heart rate may become too slow or too fast.

4. *Brachycardia.* This refers to a rate of less than 60 beats a minute (in fact, though many master athletes naturally have heartrates this slow without any ill effect), and *tachycardia* refers to a rate of more than 100 beats per minute. A rapid heart rate can damage other organs such as the brain, kidneys, lungs, or liver. And if it continues over time, tachycardia can result in *atrial fibrillation*, which is uncontrolled chaotic electrical activity in the upper chambers of the heart.

If you experience palpitations occasionally, you should, of course, tell your physician and have the problem checked out. Arrhythmias may not have to be treated if they're mild, but if they're significant enough to pose additional cardiac problems, your doctor will probably want to put you on antiarrhythmia medication. There are other options, such as electrical therapy, where the heart is "shocked" with an electrode catheter in order to change its pacing. And there is also an implantable device for patients at risk for recurrent ventricular tachycardia or fibrillation. The electrode patches have leads that are tunnelled from the heart to a small pulse generator in a pouch on the left side of the abdomen. This device serves as the metronome of the heart, giving it a regular beat.

5. *Mitral Valve Prolapse.* This condition, typical of many pre-menopausal women, is usually not serious, although it does cause symptoms that can seem alarming. Dizziness, chest pains, and palpitations can make you think that you are having a heart attack.

The mitral valve lies between the two chambers on the left side of the heart. The heart's rhythm (that typical "lub-dub" sound) is caused by the opening and closing of four valves that regulate the blood flow through the two sides of the heart. The valves open to let blood into the chamber, then shut down so that there can be no backward flow.

However, if the valve doesn't close completely, a little blood can leak backward, and if the valve is narrowed, you will hear a heart murmur or the classic mitral valve "click," a high-pitched sound of the valve leaflets snapping shut.

For years, this condition was thought to be psychosomatic—that only nervous, high-strung women suffered from these symptoms. But since the advent of new diagnostic techniques, it's clear that this is no imaginary problem. Physicians now routinely do an exercise stress test, sometimes with a thallium dye to measure the blood flow through the valve; an EKG or electrocardiogram; or an echocardiogram, which produces a picture with sound waves similar to a sonagram and gives a good image of the structure of the heart.

Most women never need treatment for this condition. However, if palpitations continue and are very disturbing, your doctor may prescribe antiarrhythmia drugs. The only danger of mitral valve prolapse is that it puts you at greater risk for *bacterial endocarditis,* an infection of the mitral valve leaflets. Preventive antibiotics are sometimes prescribed for women with MVP who are going to have a surgical procedure that might leave them vulnerable to bacterial infections.

6. *Syndrome* X. This syndrome is particular to women, and is a very frustrating problem for many cardiologists who may come up with completely normal tests on women who continually complain of excruciating heart pain.

The women who have Syndrome X don't have problems with their large blood vessels but, rather, with the microscopic interior vessels. They may have an extreme hypersensitivity in the nerves leading to the heart, esophagus, and chest. It is thought that much of the problem is due to a hormone imbalance and, in fact, estrogen replacement generally relieves the symptoms.

7. *Stroke.* A stroke occurs when a blood vessel that carries oxygen to the brain bursts or is clogged by a blood clot. Without oxygen, nerve cells to the affected area die and the part of the body controlled by those cells loses function. We're born with all the nerve cells we'll ever have and can't manufacture any more, so if many of them are killed off at once, we can suffer a great deal of impairment. Luckily, the brain is very flexible and is often able to compensate for loss of function by having another portion of the brain take over.

The two halves of the brain, the right and left hemispheres, are connected by a fibrous band called the *corpus callosum*, which is better developed in women than in men. Women tend to use both sides of the brain simultaneously for tasks that men tend to accomplish with more dependence on only one side. So even if a woman loses a bit of function from the left side of her brain, a corresponding right-side area may be more likely able to take over. This is why physical therapy and speech therapy are often more successful in women than in men.

## Is Medication Necessary for All Women with Heart Disease?

Doctors used to believe that some people simply had high cholesterol that could not be managed by diet and exercise and that, in order to protect the heart, it was necessary to give cholesterol-lowering drugs.

However, a review of the medical literature indicates that these drugs have little substantial effect on improving life expectancy or reducing deaths from heart attack, according to a report by Dr. Allan Brett in the Sept., 1989, issue of the *New England Journal of Medicine*.

It's interesting to look at two studies on these drugs (one on *cholestyramine* or *Questran* and one on *gemifibrozil* or *Lopid*) that were conducted at the Lipid Research Clinics Trial (1984) and in the Helsinki Heart Study (1987). Only 1 or 2 percent of those treated actually benefited from these drugs. It was clear that although cholesterol plays some part in the heart disease story, there are many other players as well.

Reducing fat and cholesterol in the diet, taking vitamin and mineral supplements, eliminating cigarettes and reducing alcohol, exercising daily and managing stress appear to be the most important preventive-care strategies.

The same is true of blood pressure medication. Although anti-hypertensive drugs will lower pressure, you only continue to benefit as long as you take the drugs. Do you really see yourself taking a hypertension pill every single day for the rest of your life? The large-scale study of 612 individuals in Helsinki, Finland revealed that although the drugs did offer a 35 percent reduction in blood pressure, "The participants developed twice as much heart disease after five years when compared to a control group of patients that took fewer hypertensive and cholesterol-lowering drugs."

Don't rely on medications only to do the work you need to do with your own preventive care tactics. You can effect a huge change in your heart profile by following the Ryback Heart Disease Prevention Plan.

## THE RYBACK HEART DISEASE PREVENTION PLAN

You don't need to depend on medication or surgery to help your heart (except for extreme cases, of course). You can lose weight if you're overweight, lower your cholesterol, manage your stress more effectively, stop smoking, get treatment for your high blood pressure, and maintain a regular exercise regimen that will protect your heart. And you can work closely in coordination with your doctor to get the kind of treatment you need.

### How to Eat Right to Keep Your Heart Young

For a healthy heart, you should be eating something from every food group. You should have lots of complex carbohydrates like bread, pasta, cereals, a good amount of vegetables and legumes (beans and peas), a healthy amount of fruits, and just a little fish, chicken, and, very occasionally, meat, as well as small amounts of fat-free milk, cheese, and yogurt. You can add in a very small amount of oil for cooking as well. The most important recommendation is: keep your fats as low as you possibly can, from 10 to 20 percent of your daily caloric intake.

Everything you ingest has to pass through your bloodstream. And your bloodstream, obviously, also helps to feed your heart. The blood from your veins is pumped through the lungs to be oxygenated and returned to the body via the arterial network. This means that anything carried in the blood may deposit on the inside walls of the arteries, causing a buildup of plaque. Heart disease progresses slowly, over many years. By the time we reach adulthood, the plaque build-up may close off arterial passages by as much as 65 percent, and a few more percentage points may push us over the edge to a heart attack.

The more fat we eat, and the more cholesterol we eat and manufacture on our own, the more opportunity for our heart's arteries to become clogged. The more fiber, vegetables, and fruits we ingest, the more likely our heart will function well and smoothly both now, and for years to come.

We cannot eliminate fat from our diet entirely (although if we cut our fat consumption in half, we'd be in great shape). We have a strong craving for fat because we depend on it for survival. Our ancestors, thousands and thousands of years ago, were able to survive best when they had the most fat storage, for the energy they needed to catch their prey and run away from wild animals during periods of famine. Today, we have to ingest just a little fat for storage, mainly for protection and padding for all our body's organs.

## ALL ABOUT DIETARY FATS

Saturated fats are solid at room temperature; unsaturated and monosaturated fats tend to be more liquid. Saturated fats are found in red meat (which is larded with animal fat) and in dairy products. They're also found in products that contain coconut or palm oil—most crackers, cookies and fast foods are unfortunately loaded with these oils. The more saturated fat we consume, the more damage we can do to our heart.

Americans eat between 30 and 40 percent of their daily diet in fat, which is nearly twice what they should be getting. The fats you do consume should be mainly mono- and polyunsaturated fats.

Butter and lard are saturated; margarine is polyunsaturated. However, because of the harmful transfatty acids that are produced when liquid margarine is hydrogenated so that it can stand up on bread, you're not helping your heart any. Instead, dip your bread in olive oil—or eat it dry. You can cook with olive, canola, or peanut oil.

So how much fat in your diet is advisable? A variety of studies have been done using 30 percent fat or 20 percent fat diets on individuals with heart disease. None of these have shown dramatic improvements whether with blood cholesterol reduction, with prevention of second heart attacks, or with longevity after a first heart attack.

However, very impressive results were obtained by Dr. Dean Ornish, who has been able to reverse heart disease in many patients by putting them on a 10-percent-fat diet in combination with a daily exercise program and daily participation in yoga, meditation, and group support meetings. The individuals in his program at the University of California at San Francisco ate a vegetarian diet with very little oil. After one year, eighteen of the twenty-two experimental subjects (82 percent) showed a reduction of heart blockage, while two-thirds of the control group of nineteen subjects showed deterioration and the rest showed no change.

Can you do it? Can you really stick to such a rigorous eating plan? Most individuals aren't that motivated, and find that the switch to shopping, cooking, and eating in a totally different way is extremely challenging to maintain.

My suggestion is that you strive to lower your fat consumption a little each month until you're down to 20 percent. If you feel wonderful and you're highly motivated, you can keep going lower. However, you must remember that what you eat is just a part of your entire plan for renovating your heart. Each element of treatment or prevention contributes its own significant part.

## GOOD CHOLESTEROL VS. BAD CHOLESTEROL

Cholesterol is not a fat but rather a biochemical alcohol that functions as a transport mechanism. When we eat saturated fat, we raise our "bad" or LDL cholesterol level by stimulating our liver to manufacture cholesterol and to deliver it into the bloodstream. We need a certain amount of it to survive, but we don't have to eat much of it, since the body produces cholesterol on its own.

After you digest the excess fat in a food product and your liver has processed it, it's delivered throughout the body by *very low-density lipoproteins*, or VLDLs. Once they've delivered the fat, they become LDLs and can begin to harden on the inside of artery walls.

The "good" cholesterol can in some ways salvage this situation. These HDL or high density lipoproteins are able to pull plaque away from artery walls and bring it back to the liver to be recycled or broken down and excreted.

Even though it's unclear as to whether you can undo cholesterol damage solely with a fat-free diet, it's definitely clear that you can prevent further damage if you change some of your habits. You may not be able to get the plaque deposits off your artery walls with only proper nutrition, but you can certainly reduce the level of cholesterol currently floating around in your blood.

For every percentage point that you can lower your blood cholesterol level, you can decrease your risk of heart disease by two percent. That's a 2-for-1 payoff—not bad!

## EAT LESS FOR A STRONGER HEART

Eating three meals a day is convenient, but it's not the best idea for living ten years longer. According to a study done at the University of Toronto in Canada, cholesterol can be maintained better when we eat more small meals throughout the day—when we "graze" like cows rather than sit down to a groaning board. When we eat large meals and bump up our blood sugar, our pancreas has to create more insulin in order to balance the glucose levels in the blood. This in turn stimulates the production of an enzyme that increases cholesterol production by the liver. The study showed that those eating smaller, more frequent meals had fewer peaks and valleys in their blood sugar levels. This meant that they saw their insulin levels drop by 28 percent, their total cholesterol by 8.5 percent and their LDL cholesterol by 13.5 percent.

It's not such a bad idea to reduce total food intake if you're thinking about living ten years longer. Dr. Roy Walford, one of the pioneers of nutrition as a longevity booster and a participant in the

Biosphere II experiment, has shown that dietary restriction in rats both enhances their immune system and reduces the incidence of age-related diseases. Dr. Walford and his colleagues are now practicing what he preaches and have reduced their daily caloric consumption drastically in an attempt to live to 120.

## CHOOSING NATURAL FOODS, NOT PROCESSED FOODS

We've all been swayed by commercial advertising that promises cholesterol-free products. But remember, just because they aren't adding cholesterol doesn't mean they haven't put in the fat—which can create cholesterol as soon as we eat it.

Even fat-free products have their drawbacks. In order to keep flavor in a cookie or cracker, something has to be added when fat is subtracted—and that something is usually empty calories in the form of sugar. Read the labels carefully on all boxes on your supermarket shelf because no one has yet developed a way to process food and give you all the vitamins and minerals you need minus the fats, salt, and calories. That goes particularly for the processed meats in the deli counter, most of which are about 70 percent fat.

So what should you eat? Watch out for anything in a fancy box. For any packaged food, choose those such as a grain or bean that have only that product and nothing else inside. Fruits and vegetables, grains and cereals are your best choices for a heart-healthy diet. Fresh fish is also beneficial, especially those deep-water fishes like salmon, trout, kipper, herring, and sardines, which are high in omega-3 fatty acids. These good fats appear to inhibit clotting and open the tight pathways of the arteries. Less blood stickiness and wider arteries mean a reduction in your risk for heart attack.

A study using omega-3s for patients undergoing *angioplasty* (a procedure where a tiny balloon is used to open the narrowing in the arterial wall) found that those patients who had 3.2 grams of omega-3s per day in the form of fish-oil capsules had half as many recurrences of arterial blockage as those who did not have the omega-3s.

# THE FIBER CONNECTION

Fiber is not just good for your gastrointestinal system, but will also protect your heart. It's a complex carbohydrate that isn't broken down by the digestive enzymes but, rather, moves through the intestinal tract, carrying water with it. It's only found in plant cells, and generally, Americans don't eat enough of it.

There are two types of fiber—*soluble* and *insoluble fiber*. Soluble fiber, which is found in oatmeal, oat bran, barley, seeds and most beans, dissolves in water.

Insoluble fiber doesn't dissolve in water. It works in the intestinal tract to promote prompt elimination. This fiber, while not much protection against heart disease because it doesn't affect cholesterol levels, is definitely beneficial to the intestines and can help to prevent colon cancer. Wheat bran, whole grain products and most vegetables contain insoluble fiber.

Start with a goal of 20 grams of soluble plus insoluble fiber a day, and gradually increase to 30. It will make a big difference in your general health picture.

# IS VEGETARIANISM FOR YOU?

If you ate only fruit, vegetables and grains, you would have ample protein to keep you healthy and strong. If, on a particular day, you consumed two servings of carrots, two of summer squash, a cantaloupe, two apples, and a dish of beans and rice, with a piece of whole grain bread at each meal, you'd be getting as much protein as you usually consume when you eat fish or fowl. The vitamins and minerals you'd be ingesting would be protective to your heart, and you would also be reaping the benefits of low-fat eating without resorting to any processed food whatsoever. Vegetarians have lower cholesterol and blood pressure, due to the higher levels of minerals—magnesium, calcium and potassium—in their diets.

Many Seventh Day Adventists maintain a vegetarian lifestyle and have been studied for their excellent health. Women in this group tend to live seven and a half years longer than the national norm and also have a lower incidence of most forms of cancer. The death rate due to heart disease is about half that of the general American population.

You don't have to become a total vegetarian in order to live ten years longer. Rather, you may want to emulate their general style of eating: fresh, unprocessed foods, high in complex carbohydrates and fiber, and low in fat, sugar, and salt. This type of eating will keep your weight down as well—a steamy baked potato with a little malt vinegar and chives is only 100 calories. Turn that same potato into French fries (300 calories) or potato chips (800 calories), and you've effectively reduced your lifespan.

The closer to a food's natural state the better. So wash it, cut it and steam or bake it, and you'll be doing fine.

# WHAT ABOUT VITAMINS AND MINERALS?

The amount of minerals in your diet can affect your blood pressure. And the minerals you ingest have a lot to do with how low you can keep that pressure. High blood pressure lays the groundwork for atherosclerosis by damaging the arterial walls and the heart muscle itself. So to keep it low by eating well, consider the following four items:

## 1. Keep Dietary Sodium Low

The body has built-in mechanisms for ridding the body of salt, however, it does pay a price for this intricate dance of minerals and water. When you ingest sodium, your brain signals your kidneys to excrete or retain as much as is needed. As the kidneys are challenged by too much salt, blood volume is increased and, therefore, pressure increases too.

Postmenopausal women with high blood pressure are three times more likely to suffer a heart attack and seven times more likely to have a stroke—and this can shorten their lives by as much as ten to twenty years. This means that it's additionally important for women to watch the sodium in their diets.

The INTERSALT study, an international survey of over 10,000 individuals in 52 centers representing 32 countries, has discovered a strong relationship between high-sodium diets and hypertension. In centers where sodium intake was high, 13.4 percent of those tabulated were hypertensive, as opposed to just 1.7 percent in countries where sodium intake was low.

A good rule of thumb is to omit salt on the table and use it sparingly to taste in cooking, if at all. Another tip is to avoid foods with hidden salt—virtually anything processed, such as TV dinners, canned soup, deli meats and commercial ketchup and mustard. It goes without saying that fast food is salt-saturated. A McDonald's Big Mac has 950 mg. of sodium and a Burger King Whopper with cheese has a whopping 1,164 mg. of sodium. Anyone at risk for heart disease should be consuming no more than 1,500 mg. per day! So stick with natural foods that you cook yourself in order to regulate salt.

### 2. Keep Dietary Potassium High

Potassium is the counterpart to salt in the body. There's a lot of sodium in the plasma around each cell and very little potassium; inside the cell, there's lots of potassium and little sodium. Potassium acts in some to lower blood pressure.

A research project at the Temple Univerisity School of Medicine in Philadephia took ten individuals with normal blood pressure and fed them two different diets; half had a high potassium diet, and half had a low potassium diet. They all consumed the same amount of sodium. After just nine days, the diastolic blood pressure of the low potassium group rose from 91 to 95; sodium and fluid retention also rose.

This study indicates that the better balance we can achieve between potassium and sodium, the more we'll be able to regulate our blood pressure and keep it on an even keel. Dr. James Scala, author of *High Blood Pressure Relief Diet*, suggests that we keep our potassium to sodium balance in a 3 to 1 ratio. Since natural, un-processed foods contain more potassium than sodium, and animal products and processed foods contain more sodium than potassium, it's not difficult to figure out what to buy and eat for better blood pressure. Just stay on the side of your supermarket where nothing comes in a box: Potassium, happily, is present in many natural foods—bananas, tomatoes, dates, lima beans, squash, and pota-toes.

## 3. Keep Dietary Calcium and Magnesium High

These two minerals, as you recall from Chapter Seven, help to keep your bones strong. But interestingly enough, they also help to keep your blood vessels elastic and flexible. Blood pressure goes up when arteries narrow, building up resistance to the flow of blood. But when muscle cells relax, so do arterial walls. Calcium plays a big part in relaxing the muscles in the arteries, so it helps in regulating blood pressure. Calcium can be found in dairy products (which should be low-fat, of course), green leafy vegetables, fish with bones (mackerel, blue fish, salmon in the can), broccoli, spinach, and soy products.

Magnesium is similar to calcium in its various functions; you need about half as much of this mineral as you do calcium. Although, on its own, it has not been shown to lower blood pressure, it is use-ful for heart attack patients and those undergoing heart surgery because it apparently regulates heart rhythm, preventing arrthymias that might start up under the trauma of a cardiac event or surgery. The best sources of magnesium are whole grains, legumes, seafood, soy products, nuts, green leafy vegetables, apricots, and bananas.

## 4. Ingest Enough Niacin (Vitamin B₃)

This interesting vitamin has been found to raise HDL and lower LDL cholesterol at high dosage, and it's an inexpensive tool in the battle for a healthier heart, costing only $50 for a year's supply. It is water soluble, like other B vitamins. When taken in large doses—about 25 to 150 times greater than a normal vitamin dosage—this vitamin becomes a drug that reduces the amount of LDLs produced by the liver and also reduces the liver's synthesis of triglycerides. In addition, it slows down the rate by which HDLs are removed from the blood.

Unfortunately, in the massive doses of 1,500 to 3,000 mg. a day needed for niacin to have this result, it has been found to have unpleasant side-effects. Many patients complain of a niacin "flush," and some complain of itching, headaches, heartburn, nausea and gastrointestinal distress. There have been a few reports of toxic reactions to niacin; it can cause hepatitis. (Apparently the timed-release formulas are the culprits because they stay in the blood long enough to disturb the function of liver enzymes.) Niacin can also elevate blood sugar levels and may bring on symptoms of diabetes in some patients. It can also cause peptic ulcers or intestinal bleeding.

For these reasons, it must be taken with care and with your physician's approval, and only after you have found that rigorous attention to diet and exercise alone aren't lowering your cholesterol levels. You can reduce some of the side-effects by taking an aspirin about half an hour prior to the niacin.

— SIDEBAR I —

### A COMPARISON OF LOVASTATIN AND NIACIN (VITAMIN B₃)

Niacin, when taken under a doctor's supervision, may be as effective in lowering cholesterol as the medication *lovastatin*. It's much less expensive and has fewer side-effects.

A comparison of the two revealed that while the medication is more effective at lowering overall cholesterol levels, niacin is better at raising HDL cholesterol. Both are equally good at decreasing triglyceride levels.

## GOOD EATING TIPS

1. Don't scrap your old eating habits entirely. Just change the proportion of foods on your plate. Instead of making meat or chicken your main course, use them as a condiment and let them flavor the rice, beans, barley, and vegetables that will now become the stars of your meal.

2. Stir frying is a great way to introduce yourself to new, heart-healthy vegetables. If you're not sure you're going to like swiss chard and triticale, combine them in a wok with some other vegetables and grains you already know and enjoy.

3. If you get bored with fresh fruit as a dessert, dress it up. You can put diced pears in half a cantaloupe and sprinkle with raisins and walnuts. You can try kumquats in a bowl of strawberries and blueberries, dressed with a splash of grapefruit juice. Use your imagination for exciting combinations.

4. Substitute soy cheese for real cheese to cut fat and add dietary estrogens. Soy cheese, found at most health food stores, can be tucked inside a steamed potato with sweet basil and dill.

5. Get rid of prepared salad dressings and make your own from different vinegars and a little olive oil. You can add chives, rosemary, dill, or thyme to the vinegar to flavor it differently each time.

## How to Exercise to Keep Your Heart Strong

Getting up a little earlier in the morning to take a brisk, two-mile walk can save you from a heart attack. It's easy, costs nothing and can become a good habit you can enjoy every day. If you're having trouble making a commitment to getting into good shape, review Chapter 3 for details on creating an easy, enjoyable activity program you can incorporate into your busy life.

Exercise is a triple-threat to atherosclerosis: it raises HDL cholesterol and lowers LDL cholesterol and triglycerides; it provides elasticity for arterial walls; and it improves the blood clotting system. Daily activity that gets the heart pumping makes the blood less thick so that it flows better. The heart itself—which is a muscle—is strengthened each time you go out to bat a ball or jog around the neighborhood. When you're resting, the heart pumps about five quarts of blood per minute, but during exercise, it takes on about 20 quarts per minute. You need to work at an aerobic level that improves the pumping action of the heart. Under stress, the heart contracts more powerfully and then, during relaxation, it recovers more quickly. This means that you are effectively training your heart to be more efficient. A heart that's in good shape can do more work for longer periods of time. You have to use it or lose it!

There are other benefits to daily activity. Women who exercise are less likely to be obese, to develop diabetes, to be hypertensive or to suffer from stress. Their sex lives improve, their mental faculties become more acute and aware, and they tend to require less medication overall.

In a study of over 500 postmenopausal women, it was found that adding just 300 kilocalories of exercise per week (that's about three extra 25-minute walks) helped them enormously over a three-year period. Unlike their sedentary colleagues, they didn't experience the same physical or mental declines; their weight stayed on target as did their HDL cholesterol. These women showed a 48 percent lower death rate over the three years of the study than those women who didn't exercise.

You don't have to be a marathoner to improve your heart. You need the four parameters of good activity: *fitness, flexibility, endurance* and *muscle strength*. And those elements will come in a well-rounded program that includes aerobic exercise (walking, jogging, swimming, racquet sports, dance, step training) as well as non-aerobic exercise (yoga, tai chi, moderate weight training). (See Chapter Three for a full discussion of exercise.)

In order to get aerobic benefit for your heart, you must get your heart rate up to about 70 percent of its maximum capacity. You can do this by following this formula:

220 – your age × 70 percent = maximum rate.

If you're now 40, the formula reads:

220 – 40 × 70 percent = 126.

During your workouts, you need time to stretch out and build slowly to your maximum, and then, after about twenty minutes of working hard, you need to cool down so that your pulse slowly returns to normal.

Before you begin any exercise program, check with your physician to be certain your particular plan is right for your general state of health. Then get yourself a good pair of walking or cross-training shoes, set your alarm clock for twenty minutes or half an hour earlier in the morning, and get started. You have nothing to lose but your LDLs!

## Easy Lifestyle Changes to Protect Your Heart

There's no question about it: You have to stop smoking if you want a healthy heart. Nicotine raises blood pressure; toxins damage artery walls. Smoking can cause blood clots and constrict blood vessels throughout the body, making it harder for blood to flow freely. Smoking also has an adverse effect on your mental health, since you get less oxygen flow to your brain cells when you puff on a cigarette. If you don't think as clearly, it's harder to discipline yourself to maintain an excellent diet and exercise program so that your heart can reap the benefits.

Cutting down on excess alcohol is also an important step to take. It's been shown, particularly in studies on French red-wine drinkers, that a little alcohol protects the heart by increasing HDLs. These take cholesterol away from the plaque deposits so that they can be removed from the blood by the liver. Red wine also inhibits platelet activation and may interfere with blood clotting—one vital trigger for heart attack.

But too much of a good thing turns the picture around. Heavy drinking can damage the heart muscle and bring on congestive heart failure. If you consume one or two drinks a day, that's fine. (Those drinks should be made up of six no more than ounces of wine, twelve ounces of beer or one ounce of hard liquor). But beyond that, you may be setting the scene for arrhythmias, hypertension, strokes and brain hemorrhage.

If you're a ten-cup-a-day coffee drinker, (and particularly if you grab a cup of coffee instead of preparing a healthy breakfast or lunch), it's time to make some changes. Although two or three cups of daily caffeine won't hurt your heart, excess caffeine raises heart rate and blood pressure and may give you the "jitters." Remember, everything in moderation.

## Stress Reduction for a Better Heart

Do you worry a lot? If you're constantly anxious and always on edge, if you find it difficult to relax, you are producing the stress hormones that can, over time, damage your heart.

When you are under pressure constantly, you are always in the "fight or flight" pattern where your stomach is tied in knots, your head pounds, and your arteries constrict. Prolonged stress without end keeps that alarm switch in your body in a constant "on" position.

The brain alerts the body to anxiety or danger, and the adrenal glands pump out the stress hormones *adrenalin, noradrenalin,* and *cortisol.* These in turn raise LDL levels and may cause negative changes in the blood vessels. When you're always under pressure, your arteries are always constricted, and blood clots can form which can lead to heart attack or stroke. (See Chapter Four for a full discussion of the stress cycle.)

Women play so many roles in their lives and often load one responsibility on top of another, insisting that they can handle them all. Some women tend to deal poorly with stress and can often try to cover their inability to cope with excesses of other kinds, like going without sleep, smoking cigarettes, or abusing alcohol or recreational drugs.

When you learn ways to deal with stress, you can work to change your reactions and protect your heart. You'll also feel better when you're in control.

Dr. Dean Ornish, head of the Preventive Medicine Research Institute in Sausalito, CA, is the first medical doctor to acknowledge that in order to reverse heart disease, we must heal the mind as well as the body. Through his active work and perseverance, he has convinced insurance companies that individuals pursuing good health should be reimbursed for care that involves not only medication or surgery, but diet, exercise, meditation, and a change of attitude as well.

Dr. Ornish, Dr. James Lynch and others explain that heart disease is often a symptom of a larger disease—that of isolation and loneliness. People can, in fact, die of a broken heart. But Ornish states, "Conversely, anything that leads to real intimacy and feelings of connection can be healing in the real sense of the word: to bring together, to make whole." He discusses intimacy as either "horizontal" or "vertical." *Horizontal intimacy* occurs through support groups; *vertical intimacy* you can give to yourself alone through meditation and prayer.

His findings were confirmed by others in three large-scale studies involving almost 7,000 people in Alameda County, California; over 2,000 subjects in Evans County, Georgia; and over 13,000 individuals in Eastern Finland. Those who were socially isolated (independent of other cardiac risk factors such as cholesterol and blood pressure levels) were two to three times likelier to die of heart disease than those who had strong emotional ties with others.

Women are typically more prone to this type of stress in later life. According to Dr. Lynda Powell of the Yale School of Medicine, men handle their stress by ranting and raving: however women tend to keep it all inside—they are more likely to experience distress in the form of loneliness and despair. There is often a coverup for feelings of anger and resentment which, as we know, can trigger the production of stress hormones. Over time, the consequences of mind and body take their toll on the heart.

When someone says to you, "Take it easy, just relax," don't just nod and agree that you will when you know you really won't. Relaxation is just as important a form of holistic medicine as a good diet or exercise program. It should be easy to relax, but many women find it virtually impossible. Some women are used to being tense all the time, they have no idea what a calm mind and an easy, comfortable body feels like. The best way to overcome this is to learn relaxation techniques. These can't be mastered in one day—they must become an integral part of your life in order for them to make a difference.

## MEDITATION AND PRAYER

Meditation (see Chapter 4) is many things to many people, but basically it involves sitting quietly and clearing the mind of distraction. You can concentrate on your breathing, or on one word such as "peace" or "calm." In order to have a beneficial effect on the heart, meditation must be practiced conscientiously and mindfully. Once you have become accustomed to sitting and breathing, you can add more healing techniques, such as visualizing the blood through your circulatory system, cleaning it out, and making it flow smoothly. Visualize any plaque deposits on the inside of your artery walls breaking up into tiny particles and being swept away.

1. *Looking out for yourself.* Be greedy about your time alone—don't let other obligations keep you from your daily meditation. This is *your* time to protect your heart. Many women have trouble saying "no" and take on every imaginable type of favor, if asked. It's nice to feel wanted, but if you're overwhelmed by doing everyone else's job, including

your own, you may build up a lot of inner rage about being so put upon. Instead, make a space for yourself in your world, and be sure that you are fulfilling your own needs before you tackle anyone (or everyone) else's.

2. *Developing a social support group.* It's vital that you have friends and family around you if you want to live to a ripe old age. In other cultures, older people are revered and honored as heads of the household. You become *more* valuable in these societies as you age. Unfortunately, we are not yet that enlightened in North America and have to create our own "extended families" to rally around us.

If your spouse is no longer living (women typically outlive their husbands by about six years) and your children have moved across the country, it's vital that you surround yourself with people who care. Join a variety of clubs and groups; start a weekly meeting group to discuss women's issues at your church or synagogue; take on responsibility for gathering together the important women in your life. United, there is nothing you cannot do—including taking a positive stand against heart disease.

## Being a Heart-healthy Woman

It doesn't matter how old you are now, or whether you're completely healthy. It's still important for you to maintain a preventive heart-care program, because this illness is an insidious, slowly growing condition that can rob you of many valuable years.

If we get in the swing of keeping up with our resolutions to eat better, exercise more and take time to smell the roses and relax, we can extend our lifespan. A conscientious program of good heart health will make the difference.

So many women live beyond the age of 85 in poor health, confined to nursing homes or kept home-bound by fatigue and chronic illness. We want to stop that pattern, and make every day of our lives count.

Your heart must keep pumping, over and over, throughout your life. Why not make every beat of your heart a strong, loud one, proclaiming to the world that you're ready for ten extra years of excellent health?

# STOP SMOKING
## AND ADD YEARS TO YOUR LIFE

## CHAPTER 10

"I was usually photographed as a fresh-faced girl with a cigarette in her hand," said Janet Sackman, known back in the '40s as the pretty and glamorous "Lucky Strike Cover Girl." But now in her mid-60s, Ms. Sackman spoke without her larynx. It had been removed as a result of smoking over a 33-year period.

In the prime of his life, at the age of 38, Dr. Sigmund Freud was frightened by the irregular heartbeats he felt in his chest. He consulted his own physician, and was advised to give up his smoking habit. This great healer of the human psyche did so, of course, and had this to say about it:

> There were tolerable days. . . . Then came suddenly a severe
> affectation of the heart, worse than I ever had when smoking. . . .
> And with it an oppression of mood in which images of dying and
> farewell scenes replaced the more usual fantasies. . . . It is
> annoying for a doctor who has to be concerned all day long with
> neurosis, not to know whether he is suffering from a justifiable or
> hypochondriacal depression.

And as you might suspect, Dr. Freud yielded to his human frailties and succumbed to smoking once again—twenty cigars a day. And continued, except for one 14-month abstention, for the rest of his life, despite the fact that he admitted that it interfered with his studies.

By age 67, Freud developed cancer in his mouth and jaw. Thirty-three operations later, he continued to smoke until he actually lost his jaw. The artificial jaw caused him much pain and made it very difficult for him to swallow. He remained addicted to smoking right up to his cancer-induced death.

Freud was undeniably a brilliant individual. He mastered the workings of the human mind. He was skilled at hypnosis. He was well trained in medicine and biology. Yet this physician was not able to heal his own smoking addiction. He failed, and did not learn from his own failings in this particular area of behavior.

Today there is a difference, thanks in large part to a number of women who have helped change the public's perception of smoking. In 1954, Eva Cooper sued the R.J. Reynolds Tobacco Co. for contributing to her husband's death due to cancer. The court ruled that there was insufficient evidence to prove that the Camels her husband smoked caused his illness.

In 1968, the Philip Morris Co. introduced Virginia Slims, the first cigarette designed for women. But women who valued their health fought back. Within a decade, a court-ordered injunction prohibiting smoking in her office was won by Donna Shrimp of New Jersey. By 1983, San Francisco passed the country's first strong work-place anti-smoking ordinance.

In 1988, smoking was banned on domestic flights of less than two hours. By 1994, another brave woman took up the banner against smoking; former U.S. Surgeon General Joycelyn Elders spoke up for government regulation of cigarettes. The tide was finally beginning to turn.

At this time, the FDA was considering reclassifying tobacco as a drug. The Labor Dept proposed prohibiting smoking in all indoor workplaces, and a class-action lawsuit was filed in New Orleans against six tobacco companies for deceiving the public.

Today a body of knowledge exists that allows us to learn from our failings. This body of knowledge informs us of the specific chemistry of the biological damage of smoking: the statistics that link smoking to cancer, emphysema, heart disease, cholesterol build-up; the biological and psychological consequences of quitting once you're addicted; and, finally, what methods work best, which "quitting technologies" have the best track record. In this chapter, we'll take a look at all this. So that if you fail, you can learn from your failure and start again.

Although the overall rate of smoking has dropped from 40 percent to about 25 percent in the past three decades, the rate for women increased three-fold in the three decades prior to 1965, and has only gone down by about 10 percent since then. In addition, women are likely to start smoking at an earlier age than men, and are less likely to quit than men.

Though it's crystal clear that smoking is hazardous to your health, most doctors don't concern themselves with dissuading their patients from smoking, possibly because they know how difficult it is to do so. A study by Dr. Erica Frank has revealed that only about half the smokers surveyed had ever been told by their physicians to stop smoking, for instance.

Smoking is particularly harmful to pregnant women, and more particularly, to their unborn babies. Babies born to smokers are, on the average, seven ounces lighter and one-half inch shorter than babies born to mothers who didn't smoke. Even more serious, they're more likely to suffer from birth defects and learning disabilities.

Quitting smoking is not easy: even more so for women than for men, it appears. But with the help of this chapter, you'll be able to quit if you persist. Although only about 1 in 5 are able to quit on their first try, my program makes allowance for that and assures you that if you try again and learn from your failures, you'll eventually be able to master this nasty habit and add years to your life.

## PERSISTENCE LEADS TO SUCCESS

The bad news is that of all who are successful at quitting, as many as 80 percent will suffer relapse. The good news is that those women who learn from their first fall from grace will be more successful the next time around. The great news is that, for those who persist, and recognize failure as a learning path to greater chances of success the next time around, success is virtually guaranteed. Unfortunately, Freud didn't know this. Had this information been available, I'm certain he would have avoided the excruciating pain of jaw cancer which afflicted his final years. He might even have lived longer.

The process of quitting smoking is a circular path—actually more like a circular coil. The ultimate goal—being smoke-free—is in the center. We start at the outer edge and work our way to the center. It takes four steps to go around the circle once. Every time we complete a revolution we get closer to the center, the goal. If you're among the lucky 20 percent who can do it first time around, then there's only one coil in your circle. If it takes you five falls from grace, then there are five coils in your circle.

The four steps to complete each revolution are as follows:

**Denial ⟶ Conflict ⟶ Action ⟶ Change**

### 1. Overcome Your Denial

Half the struggle of quitting smoking then, is overcoming the denial that smoking is a form of systematic suicide and getting through the conflict of being responsible for making your life both shorter as well as miserable except for the immediate gratification of smoking.

### 2. Making the Decision—the Key to Success

When a smoker comes to my office to discuss quitting, she's already into the second step, *Conflict*. Thank goodness, I don't have to deal with her *Denial*. That's already been taken care of by her spouse, her family doctor, or certain excruciating pains in her chest. Increasingly, I'm happy to add, the workplace is becoming more involved in that process of encouraging smoke-free environments. So she comes into my office and asks: "Dr. Ryback, can you make me quit smoking?"

"No!" I retort adamantly. "I refuse to treat you unless *you* have made a clear and definite decision to quit. Then I'll do what I can to help you. And only then!" If she was still in *Conflict* when she sat down, by the time she arises from that chair, she's made a decision one way or another. Almost always, the decision is to quit. But it's *her* decision, not mine. And that, my dear reader, is the key to this chapter.

If you have not made a clear decision to quit, then I'll bet a hundred dollars to a dozen doughnuts (or whole wheat bagels) that you will not be successful, no matter what techniques you use, from hypnosis to having your ears stapled. On the other hand, if you've made a clear and honest decision to quit, then you will succeed.

### 3. Action to Change

So now we begin, as the psychiatrist says at the end of "Portnoy's Complaint." The Action stage begins with commitment. Once you have commitment, success is merely the follow-through. It's a matter of going through the steps of whatever technology you choose. And that technology must be integrated with some lifestyle Change, the fourth step of the cycle.

### 4. If at First You Don't Succeed

For most who go through these four steps to success and then, for whatever reason, fail, there is a whole new cycle of Denial, Conflict, Action, and Change. So it isn't easy. But with persistence, you will succeed. Each cycle gets easier; the coils get smaller as you approach the center. You learn from each cycle, you progress, and ultimately succeed.

First of all, let's define smoking addiction. According to the Diagnostic and Statistical Manual of Mental Disorders which psychiatrists and psychologists use, the diagnostic criteria for tobacco withdrawal are as follows:

1. Use of tobacco for at least several weeks at a level equivalent to more than ten cigarettes per day, with each cigarette containing at least 0.5 mg of nicotine.

2. Abrupt cessation of or reduction in tobacco use, followed within 24 hours by at least four of the following:
   a. Craving for tobacco
   b. Irritability
   c. Anxiety
   d. Difficulty in concentrating
   e. Restlessness
   f. Headache
   g. Drowsiness
   h. Gastrointestinal disturbances

Sound familiar? Isn't it nice to have a label put to it? Doesn't feel so lonely any more, does it?

# FOUR WAYS THAT SMOKING WILL KILL YOU

## 1. Cigarette "Tar"

Well, what causes all that discomfort, listed so neatly from 1 to 8? Unfortunately, the answer is neither neat nor simple. The "tar" in cigarette smoke is comprised of several thousand chemicals, including *acids, glycol, aldehydes, ketones*, as well as such corrosive and poisonous gases as *hydrogen cyanide* and *carbon monoxide*.

## 2. Carbon Monoxide Poison

Carbon monoxide comprises a relatively large 4 percent of the smoke and, once it enters the lungs, bullies its way into the red blood cells pushing aside the oxygen that would otherwise be there. This substance deprives the heart and other tissues of essential oxygen and promotes cholesterol deposits in the arteries.

## 3. Nicotine—the Poison that Seduces

The nicotine itself is a poison that initially stimulates the brain and central nervous system, but subsequently has a depressant effect on it. That's precisely why cigarettes act both as a stimulant and as a relaxant. The initial reaction is that of a picker-upper but after a few minutes, becomes quite relaxing. It is this paradoxical effect that makes smoking so desirable. It's good for what ails you, in the sense that it will stimulate you if you're bored and listless; it will relax you if you're anxious and stressed. What a great substance! If only it didn't rob you of years of life in the process.

## 4. One Hundred Fifty Thousand Cancer Deaths a Year

If that weren't bad enough, many of the components of cigarette smoke are carcinogenic. It has been argued that 30 percent of all cancer deaths can be attributed to smoking, particularly cancers of the lung, larynx, mouth, and esophagus. It also contributes to cancers of the bladder, pancreas and kidney.

Of all the cancers, the most fatal are those occurring in the lungs and pancreas. The American Cancer Society informs us that about 150,000 persons lose their lives each year because of tobacco smoking.

## Proof That Smoking Kills

In 1951, the British Medical Association sent a questionnaire on smoking habits to over 34,000 of its members. For the twenty years following, records were kept on changes in smoking habits and the causes of all deaths.

For these British doctors, the risk of dying of a heart attack before age 45 was 15 *times* greater for heavy smokers than for non-smokers. For lung cancers, respiratory diseases and strokes, the risk of death was at least *three* times as high in smokers as in nonsmokers. A whole host of other types of cancer and various diseases were just slightly correlated with smoking. Overall, you can see that the case against smoking is made quite strong by this extensive study, extensive both in terms of number of subjects and time span.

# BREATHE EASIER AND LIVE LONGER: PREVENTING HEART AND LUNG DISEASE

Lung cancer starts off very slowly. There are few symptoms until the cancer becomes very advanced. What we call "cigarette cough" has nothing to do with cancer itself; it is merely the lungs trying to get rid of the accumulated smoke deposits. It appears the self-cleaning lining of the airways is knocked unconscious or disabled by the smoke. The cilia, tiny hair-like structures which sweep the airways clean, recover overnight and try to make a clean sweep of things in the morning before they're once again knocked out by the next day's smoke. It is their feeble attempt at a clean sweep that produces "cigarette cough."

In Chapter Nine, we explored the effect of poor nutrition on atherosclerosis, the build-up of cholesterol in the arteries. Smoking is a heavy contributor to this as well. Researchers in California studied the coronary angiograms of 104 heart disease patients. Of these, 60 did not smoke and the remaining 44 continued to smoke throughout the study. After 18 months of diet and exercise, the patients were once again tested. The results showed a significant worsening of coronary artery disease in 60 percent of the vessels of the smokers, compared to only 32 percent of the vessels of the nonsmokers— almost twice as much. Apparently, smoking contributes significantly to the heart-cholesterol problem.

## Smoke Less, Live More

There is a well-known and ongoing debate between the tobacco industry and health care advocates on the smoking/lung cancer correlation. The industry claims, to this very day, that there is no *proof* that smoking leads to lung cancer. Well, technically and legally, they're right. Proof would entail *controlling* the smoking habits of a group of individuals, rather than letting them choose for themselves. That, of course, is entirely unethical. So the industry will go on claiming there is no proof, and they're technically correct.

## The Longer You Smoke, the Faster You Die

But, according to the World Health Organization, death rates are uniformly higher among smokers than among nonsmokers of both sexes. Among smokers, the death rates from all causes increase with the number of cigarettes smoked per day, the number of years the smoker has smoked, and the earlier the age at which smoking was started.

## Don't Smoke, and Add Seven Years to Your Life

So how much will smoking cessation contribute to your new-found, more becoming, and more comfortable ten years? Well, if we look at statistical averages, it appears that nonsmokers start dying off at age 72 while smokers start doing so at age 65. That is, the longevity curves for nonsmokers starts declining at 72, and for smokers at 65. By age 80, about 60 percent of nonsmokers are still alive, compared to only 30 percent of smokers.

Here's another point of view: For women between the ages of 45 and 64, the death rate due to lung cancer is four times as great for smokers as compared to nonsmokers. For those from 65 to 79, that rate is nine times higher for the smokers.

Well, tobacco industry, put that in your pipe and smoke it! But some people will never be convinced, including those in the Denial stage. They may point out, "My aunt smoked heavily all her life and never got cancer." The overall picture is quite clear, though: Women who smoke cigarettes die younger than those who don't.

## IT'S NEVER TOO LATE TO QUIT

Stopping smoking will have a very direct effect on keeping your heart healthy, especially in the advanced years. A study of over 2,500 people from 65 to 74 years of age showed that older cigarette smokers had a risk of heart disease death over 50 percent higher than that of nonsmokers and exsmokers. Even among those who had smoked for many years, quitting smoking brought heart disease risks down to nonsmoking levels within one to five years.

So if you've been smoking for years, is it too late to quit? Absolutely not! As long as cancer has not yet started, the effects of smoking are definitely reversible. According to the American Cancer Society, here's what happens once you quit:

1. Within a few days mucous in your airways breaks up and clears out of your lungs.

2. Within a few weeks, circulation improves and you will be able to smell and taste more.

3. Within a year, your risk of lung cancer begins to decrease.

In case there's any doubt about the challenge to quit smoking, let me share this very impressive piece of writing with you, by an expert on smoking.

### Why Quitting Is So Painful

First of all, quitting is not easy. According to Walter Ross, a writer on smoking for over 15 years:

When smokers first quit smoking, their heart rate slows, their blood pressure rises, and brain waves register changes. In heavily addicted smokers, temperature drops; in less-addicted smokers, it rises. All quitters do less well in coordination tests, including driving, than they did when they were smoking. Mouth ulcers are common in quitters. There are sometimes more bizarre effects.

### How to Discover the Years You'll Gain

In order to decide to quit, you need all the motivation you can get. How about living longer? We've already discussed the statistical data demonstrating a seven-year addition to your lifespan just by not smoking. To be precise however, it really depends on your age when you quit. That seven-year difference applies to the contrast between those who smoke and those who have not smoked since age 35. If you quit before age 40, you can add three years to your life. If you quit by age 50, you can add $2^1/_2$ years. If you've been smoking up to the age of 70 and quit then, you can still benefit by one additional year of life. Incidentally, this doesn't mean that if you're 70 and quit smoking, you'll live to 71. No! It means that if you quit smoking at that age, you'll live one year longer than you otherwise would, most probably somewhere in your eighties or nineties, especially if you follow my suggestions in this book.

### Are You Addicted?

First of all, let's find out if you're really addicted to smoking. You're clearly addicted if:

1. You light up within 30 minutes of awakening and that's your most satisfying cigarette of the day.

2. You smoke more than 25 high-nicotine cigarettes a day.

3. You smoke more before noon than during the rest of the day.

4. It's almost impossible to heed "no smoking" signs, as in restaurants and theaters.

If these are true for you, then it's going to be particularly rough to quit. The good news is, you *can* do it. But you'll probably have to go cold-turkey; no weaning process for you. If you're not addicted, there are some others ways to approach quitting. To find out what motivates you to smoke, take a few minutes to take the following test, developed by the National Institutes of Health.

5 = Always        2 = Seldom
4 = Usually        1 = Never
3 = Sometimes

| | | |
|---|---|---|
| A. | I smoke cigarettes to keep myself from slowing down. | 5 4 3 2 1 |
| B. | Handling and touching a cigarette is part of the enjoyment of smoking. | 5 4 3 2 1 |
| C. | I feel pleasant and relaxed when I smoke. | 5 4 3 2 1 |
| D. | I light up when I feel tense or mad about something. | 5 4 3 2 1 |
| E. | When I run out of cigarettes, I can hardly stand it until I get more. | 5 4 3 2 1 |
| F. | I smoke automatically, I am not always aware when I am smoking. | 5 4 3 2 1 |
| G. | Smoking helps me feel stimulated, turned on, creative. | 5 4 3 2 1 |
| H. | Part of my enjoyment comes in the steps I take to light up. | 5 4 3 2 1 |
| I. | For me, cigarettes are simply pleasurable. | 5 4 3 2 1 |
| J. | I light up when I feel upset or uncomfortable about something. | 5 4 3 2 1 |
| K. | I am quite aware of it when I am not smoking a cigarette. | 5 4 3 2 1 |
| L. | I may light up not realizing that I still have a cigarette in the ashtray. | 5 4 3 2 1 |
| M. | I smoke because cigarettes give me a "lift." | 5 4 3 2 1 |
| N. | Part of the pleasure of smoking is watching the smoke as I exhale. | 5 4 3 2 1 |
| O. | I want a cigarette most when I am relaxed and comfortable. | 5 4 3 2 1 |
| P. | I smoke when I am blue or want to take my mind off my worries. | 5 4 3 2 1 |
| Q. | I get "hungry" for a cigarette when I have not smoked for a while. | 5 4 3 2 1 |
| R. | I often find a cigarette in my mouth and don't remember putting it there. | 5 4 3 2 1 |

For each category below, a score of 11 or more is high, 8 to 10 is medium, and 7 or less is low.

STIMULATION CATEGORY. Total your answers to A, G, and M. If the total is more than 9, you rely on cigarettes to stimulate and enliven you, to help you work, organize, or be creative. You are a good candidate for a substitute of another kind of "high," such as five minutes of exercise in your office, or a brisk walk.

TACTILE CATEGORY. Total your answers to B, H, and N. If the total is 9 or above, an important aspect of your smoking is the feel of it. Try substituting a pen or pencil, doodling, or occupying yourself with a small toy. You may want to squeeze a tennis ball or do hand-grip exercises, or even hold a plastic cigarette.

PLEASURE CATEGORY. Total your answers to C, I, and O. A high score suggests that you are one of the people for whom cigarettes provide some real pleasure. If this is you, you are a particularly good candidate to stop because you can substitute other pleasurable outlets—reasonable eating, and social, sports, or physical activities—for smoking.

TENSION CATEGORY. Total your answers to D, J, and P. Those who score high here use tobacco as a crutch, to reduce negative feelings, and relieve problems, much like a tranquilizer. You are likely to find it easy to quit when things are going well, but staying off is harder in bad times. For you, the key is to find other activities that also work to reduce negative feelings: dancing, meditation, yoga, sports or exercise, meals, or social activities work for many such smokers.

ADDICTION CATEGORY. Total your answers to E, K, and Q. Quitting is hard for those who score high in this group because you are probably psychologically addicted and crave cigarettes. You aren't likely to succeed by tapering off gradually. Instead, try smoking more than usual for a day or two, until the craving dulls, then drop it cold turkey, and isolate yourself from cigarettes for a long period. There is good news, though: Once your craving is broken, you are less likely to relapse because you won't want to go through that distress again.

HABIT CATEGORY. Total your answers to F, L, and R. High scores indicate that you are a "reflex" smoker. For you, quitting may be relatively easy. Your goal is to break the link between smoking and your own triggering events—food, a cup of coffee, sitting down to work. Think of tapering off gradually. Each time you reach for a cigarette, stop and ask yourself out loud: "Do I really want this cigarette?" If you answer no, then skip it.

The higher your score in each category, the more that factor plays a role in your smoking. If you score low in all the categories, you probably aren't a long-term smoker. Congratulations—you have the best chance of getting off and staying off.

Combined high scores across several categories suggest that you get several kinds of rewards from smoking. For you, stopping may mean you need to try several different tactics. Being a high scorer in both *Tension* and *Addiction* is a particularly tough combination. You *can* quit—many people have—but it may be more difficult for you than for others. If you score high in *Stimulation* and *Addiction*, however, you may benefit from changing your patterns of smoking as you cut down. Smoke less often, or only smoke each cigarette partway, inhale less, use tapering filters or low-tar/nicotine brands.

### Decision and Commitment Are Key

As I mentioned earlier, there are a number of techniques to help you quit smoking. The most important thing—the "key"—is the decision and commitment. Then, having made the commitment, you can choose the technique that appeals most to you and that is available. Here are a few.

## DR. RYBACK'S NO-FAIL TEN-STEP PROGRAM TO STOP SMOKING

### 1. Supportive Environment

Get rid of all smoking paraphernalia from your home, office, and car, such as cigarettes, ashtrays, lighters. Let your friends and co-workers know in advance that you're quitting and solicit their support, so that they can offer you that rather than a cigarette, when the going gets rough. You'll find out who your real friends are.

## 2. Find a Partner

A support group would be great, but that's not always available. If you can have a buddy quit with you, it's much less lonely. At least try and have a spouse, lover, or good friend be available as a full-time support. If all three are in one person, so much the better. If you know of someone who's quit in the past year or so, search that person out as a great source of understanding and support.

## 3. Vitamin C

For the first week or so, put extra thought into having lots of fresh fruit and fruit juice. Make sure you're getting your share of vitamin C. This would be a good time to find out what your optimal dosage is.

## 4. Exercise

This is also a good time to push yourself just a little bit on your exercise routine. Your first week of quitting is a good time to push the edges of the envelope just a little bit. Whatever you do, don't get into your couch-potato mode.

## 5. Give Up Coffee for a While

I hate to break this piece of news to you, but it would really help if you give up caffeine when you first give up smoking. I know this doesn't sound very appealing if you're a coffee drinker, but it's only temporary. You see, smokers process caffeine faster, and quitting smoking returns caffeine processing to normal. Since the caffeine stays in the exsmoker's body longer than it used to, it creates a stronger case of the jitters—the last thing you need at this time. Also, you may have developed a strong habit of having a cigarette with your coffee—an extra temptation. So for those two good reasons, please forget about coffee and caffeinated soft drinks for a while.

## 6. Nicorette Gum and Skin Patches

According to a thorough review of the medical literature, the most successful approach to quitting smoking involves a combination of frequent face-to-face contact with a physician or psychologist or other professional who provides motivation and relevant information over the time period necessary to overcome the smoking habit, along with such prescription medications as Nicorette, the nicotine gum, or skin patches.

Nicorette may take a little getting used to. This gum is somewhat unfamiliar to taste, and there's a special method for chewing it which involves "parking" it in your cheek, then taking a few chews, "parking" again, and so on. But the great benefit is that you can give up your cigarettes immediately and wean yourself off the nicotine gradually. And this works!

Nicotine gum is the only proven drug treatment to help smokers quit. Nicorette, produced by Marion-Merrell Dow Pharmaceuticals of Kansas City, Missouri, is the only product of its kind currently in the United States. Your physician must prescribe it. It does not cure the urge to smoke, but it does help you get through withdrawal and deal with the irritability. In late 1991, prescribed nicotine came out in patch form under the brand names Nicoderm, Habitrol and ProStep. All you have to do is stick a patch on your upper arm and a *trans-derm process* releases nicotine through your skin gradually in tiny doses. These nicotine transdermal systems deliver nicotine through the skin in regulated doses in decreasing stages over time.

Speaking of patches, another aid to quitting is the drug Catapres (generically know as *clonidine*), whose primary function is to treat high blood pressure. But somehow, many have found a trans-derm patch of Catapres useful in overcoming the irritability and jitters that accompany quitting smoking.

## 7. Meditation with Affirmations

Find a quiet place where you definitely will not be disturbed. For 15 minutes, before breakfast and before dinner, sit quietly and comfortably with your eyes gently closed and do the following three things:

a. Repeat the affirmation, "I enjoy looking younger and living longer in a smoke-free world."

b. As you do this, picture yourself looking youthful and radiant and feeling healthy and happy.

c. If any distracting thoughts or images come up, don't get disturbed. Merely accept them into your consciousness and then say a gentle "good-bye" to them as you return to your positive imaging and affirmation. With time, you'll learn to focus more clearly and have less distractions.

As time goes by, you may want to modify the affirmation to suit your own personality and needs. Please do so. Just make sure to continue this affirmation untill you're clearly over the smoking habit.

## 8. The "Smoking Pangs" of Success

Remember the "hunger pangs of success," where hunger pangs are to be interpreted as signs of successfully becoming a thinner person? See if you can do this with smoking urges. Label urges and irritability as signs of success, as reminders that you've conquered smoking. It's a bit more challenging than the hunger pangs technique, but see if it works for you.

## 9. Dealing with Urges

Whenever you have an urge to smoke, take a few minutes out to stand (if you're sitting), take a brief walk (around the office or outdoors) and help yourself to some deep breaths of air, blowing out slowly and forcefully. If you can, take a drink of cool water. Remember, the first three days are the roughest. It starts getting easier after that.

## 10. Become a Nonsmoker

Once you decide to quit and take action, you've become a nonsmoker. So choose the nonsmoking section in restaurants and airplanes. You're now going first-class, health-wise.

## Your Taste Buds Wake Up!

Another unpleasant item I've avoided till now is weight gain. Yes, chances are you may gain two to five pounds during this process. But although that's statistically true for most, it isn't necessarily so for you. Or at least doesn't have to be. There are two major reasons you gain weight at this time. First, your taste buds and sense of smell are finally being liberated from the noxious effects of cigarette smoke. "Hallelujah!" they proclaim. "We had forgotten how good food can taste! How about some more of that linguine? And don't forget a little more of that acorn squash, while you're up. Just a smidgen of that butterscotch ice cream to top if off, thanks."

## Any Weight Gain Will Be Temporary

The second reason you may gain weight is that your metabolism may slow down temporarily once you stop smoking. So for these two reasons, you'd be wise to emphasize fresh fruits and push your exercise a bit these first couple of weeks. Even if you do gain a bit of weight, you'll most likely lose it soon if you stick to the guidelines we've discussed all along.

# WHY NONSMOKERS LOOK YOUNGER

First of all, it might be helpful to realize that in addition to the destructive effects of smoking mentioned thus far (carbon monoxide, cancer, atherosclerosis, and many other illnesses), there is one that directly affects your appearance. Smoking adversely affects circulation and as a result your skin gets less nourishment than it needs. Smokers tend to have less healthy, more wrinkled skin. By stopping smoking *now*, you can (depending on your current age) start adding one of the components of looking up to ten years younger.

In addition, those who are accustomed to smoking often have discolored fingers and nails, an unattractive characteristic which tends to add years to a woman's apparent age.

On a less permanent basis, but even more offensive to many nonsmokers, is the odor of smoke which attaches itself so readily to clothing and hair.

To this add cigarette breath, and you have a woman who has lost her appeal to many otherwise interested partners. All in all, a woman who doesn't smoke will more likely have a youthful, attractive effect on others than her counterpart who does smoke. So if you need more motivation to stop smoking, please be advised that you'll not only be physiologically younger, you'll also appear socially younger and more attractive as well.

## All Patched Up and Ready to Go!

So here you are, ready to quit. A nicotine transdermal patch on one arm, a patch of Catapres on the other. You've tossed all smoking gear, and prepared your support systems. You can still vividly recall the sickening taste of that last cigarette.

## The Whole Package: QUIT

In order to assist you in putting all this together, remember this QUIT package:

1. Question why you smoke when you know clearly that smoking:
   - ages your skin
   - results in early death
2. Understand that quitting is a personal decision to:
   - live longer
   - look younger
   - breathe easier
   - kiss sweeter
   - enjoy the flavors of food and the fragrances of flowers again
3. Initiate:
   - a support system

- a technology for quitting smoking, including patches
- an exercise program, if you haven't already
- daily affirmations

4. Treat yourself to nonsmoking accommodations in:
   - restaurants
   - airplanes
   - romantic relationships

## Persistence!

If, despite all this, you somehow don't make it the first time, it's *okay!* Don't give up. Get on the bandwagon again and go around one more revolution. You'll get through your *Denial* more quickly this time, as well as your *Conflict*. When you get to your *Action* phase, you will benefit from all you've learned the first time around. And your new *Change* mode will be even more effective.

## Your Ultimate Success Is Guaranteed

Maybe you'll make it the first time around. If not, maybe the second, or third. But one thing is guaranteed: If you don't give up, you can surely quit eventually with persistence. It gets easier with time and experience. Looking ten years younger and adding years to your life are definitely worth the effort!

— SIDEBAR I —

## SATIATION SMOKING

Satiation smoking consists of smoking your last cigarette with a vengeance. Having decided that this is your last cigarette, you make sure to inhale fully every 5 to 10 seconds until you've finished the cigarette. If you think that's fun, think again. You'll have to force yourself. You'll feel nauseated, dizzy, terrible. I don't recommend this for everyone. *Never* do it alone! Do it in the presence of your doctor. The idea is to give yourself such a sickening experience of smoking that you'll find it distasteful from then on.

— SIDEBAR II —

## DR. DAVID RYBACK
## CONTRACT TO QUIT SMOKING

I, _____, do hereby solemnly swear to quit smoking
forever.

My quitting date will be _____.

    Between now and my quitting date, I will observe my smoking behavior,
experiment with alternatives, record my urges and number of cigarettes smoked,
and keep a smoking journal. During the time I will work daily to change my smok-
ing-related thought patterns and to reduce my intake of tobacco smoke. On the
day I have chosen, I will stop smoking forever.


_____          _____
               Name                                           Date


In witness whereof:


_____          _____
       Support Person                                    Date

# THINK YOUNG
## AND BE YOUNG

$W$e were ambling along the rough footpaths atop the Hollywood hills, my mother and I, surrounded by eucalyptus and pine trees along the steep grades on either side. We were attending a small family reunion of sorts at my brother's home above Mulholland Drive, and I'd asked Mom if she'd like to go for a walk in the Hollywood hills.

We'd been walking for a good twenty minutes, chatting amiably about life and family, now walking single file along a particularly narrow path. Suddenly, I felt her hand shoving me gently. "Can't you walk a little more quickly? Why are you going so slowly?"

This, from my 80-year-old white-haired mother, despite the fact that I thought I was moving quite briskly, actually. Some women just refuse to let age determine their style. What had kept my mother so young in body and mind, I wondered. So I asked her.

"I always stay active with my social groups," she replied. "I can't stand to be with old people who sit and do nothing. I have to keep my mind active."

## AGING AND THE POWER OF THE MIND

Much of aging is in the mind. Staying young and healthy has much more to do with what goes on in the mind than what happens at a physical level. In a study of two groups of cancer patients, for instance, one with standard treatment and the other with standard treatment plus weekly support group sessions—it was found that the support group not only suffered less pain, anxiety and depression but also, quite surprisingly, lived *twice as long*. A review of the literature proves this to be consistent. Married cancer patients, for example, live longer than their unmarried counterparts.

The heart patients who were able to have their heart disease reversed (something the medical community had thought impossible till then), not only radically reduced their consumption of fat and took up physical exercise; they also formed a tight-knit support group among themselves where, with the full support of a caring doctor, they were able to unveil their deepest fears and self doubts. They talked about their fears of death, their deepest misgivings and what their lives meant to them in the final analysis. When Dr. Dean Ornish, the pioneer of this work, was asked what component of the program was most essential, he answered that none was. It was the whole enterprise of commitment to a new way of life, including not only nutrition, fitness and support groups, but also yoga, meditation and a new respect for life and loving relationships.

In my own cross-cultural research as I traveled through Europe, Asia and the Mid-east over a three-year period, I found that the healing of illness took place when two belief systems coincided—that of the healer and that of the patient. Across the various cultures, both contemporary and traditional, when a patient believed in the healing process he or she underwent and the doctor/healer/monk was also convinced of the process, then the patient got better.

The healing process seems to reside within the patient him- or herself, and just needs the permission of society, as represented through the healer, to allow the healing process to do its "magic" work. After all, the body is in the process of self-regeneration all the time, as long as the individual is alive. Some ritual, characterized by prayer, a special potion or herb, meditating on the Tao to the smell of incense, the rattling of bones or an expensive hospital stay, says to the individual's regenerative and immune processes: "Okay body, it's time for you to heal yourself. Everybody's looking at you and waiting. Drop everything else and get to work!"

This fact is well-known in our modern age and by the contemporary medical community. It's referred to as the *placebo effect*. This can best be explained by the fact that when an experiment is done and one group gets the treatment and the other doesn't, even the non-treated group improves, precisely because the group believes it's getting the treatment.

My belief is that the same can be said for the aging process. If you believe in getting old quickly, your body processes will accommodate you. You'll feel older, you'll do the things expected of an older person, and you'll give up on keeping your body young through proper nutrition and fitness and you'll look older in terms of your demeanor and your appearance.

In one sense, this book is all about gearing your *mind* to the possibilities of living longer and looking younger, even more than it is about gearing your body in that direction. As your mind goes, so will your body. Each chapter of this book engages your mind before you then engage your body.

According to the latest research, measures of mind function are even superior during the 50s and 60s than in younger years. Contrary to popular belief, the mind stays young—functioning even better through middle age—through the 50s and 60s, before it begins to decline, at least in perceptual speed and numeric skill, in the 80s. Why not make use of this increasing youthful quality of the mind to enhance a more youthful body?

In Chapter Four you learned how to use meditation and yoga to turn back the aging clock. Well, there's no limit as to how you can make use of these disciplines. The "hunger pangs of success" and the affirmations to help you become a nonsmoker are slightly different forms of meditation, in the sense that you're using your mental powers to convert a destructive habit into a constructive one. You can also use yoga and meditation to reduce stress so that your arteries start shedding the layers of cholesterol that have accumulated over the years.

Afraid of doing something as weird as yoga and meditation? Well, if you think it's more acceptable to work so hard that your increasing stress level results in open-heart surgery, then that's certainly one choice that's available to you. Frankly, I think it makes more sense to spend some time each day on such enjoyable and simple exercises than it is to give someone the permission to  cut open my rib cage and play sew-the-pieces-together with my one and only heart. Thinking young is much less expensive and not nearly as frightening.

Beyond that, would it surprise you to learn that a study of over 14,000 heart patients (the Coronary Artery Surgery Study) found that, for patients with mild angina, there is little evidence that open-heart surgery prolongs life? Neither does angioplasty, where a balloon is inserted into the arteries to squeeze away the blockages. What such surgery does do is to lessen the chest pains and discomfort that these individuals suffer, but three major studies have indicated that such surgery does *not* prolong life for these patients.

However, when you make a choice to change your lifestyle so that you take care of your body through proper nutrition, exercise, and a greater appreciation of relationships with other people, then you're choosing to take control of your life rather than signing it away to a hospital. And being in charge, feeling a sense of control over your life, is what enhances your health, strengthens your immune functions, and allows you to live out your potential lifespan, possibly into the 90s, but at least into the 80s.

## EXTENDING YOUTH: APPETITE FOR ADVENTURE

Living ten years longer is not without its psychological challenges. Even as we continue our three-times-a-week fitness routines, eat to stay slim and healthy and quit smoking, there remains a negative mystique about such a word as "aging." By definition, aging is an irreversible, inevitable change that occurs over time. We can delay its effects by ten years or so, but it is, in the end, inevitable.

And so are some of the disappointments that come with aging: a slowing down of your energy, a loss of youthful attractiveness, increasing susceptibility to illness, and seeing the aging process reflected in your close companions. Beyond looking and feeling ten years younger than your chronological age, there is an added challenge with which to come to grips. That ten-years-younger look and body offer you an alternative. The challenges of living ten years longer are undeniable. Beyond the midlife crisis, there is a mature-stage crisis, providing an opportunity for the physical and emotional, midlife regeneration.

## A Second Life to Live

Once you've made the commitment to live ten years longer, it's almost as if you have a second life to live—in terms of opportunities for a second career, a renewal of relationship, or beginning or resuming an artistic or creative calling of some sort. This "better-half adventure" can be a whole new life change in terms of values—less emphasis on physical attractiveness, a more honest approach to relationships, a greater appreciation of the spiritual as opposed to the material. Realizing the shortfall of your earlier years, you can now make up for lost time.

## The Sexual Shift

Psychiatrist Carl Jung described the "contrasexual transition" that occurs at midlife; women allow themselves to become stronger, more assertive, more self-directing. Men allow themselves to become softer and more intuitive. Both men's and women's sexuality may be freed up after the age of menopause, in that they are no longer concerned with pregnancy. Once the children have left home, the father's bread-winning role and mother's nurturing role can be abandoned in favor of less restrictive values and lifestyles. Hopefully, the couple can stay in tune with one another despite the transformations. And quite possibly, the sex roles may be less stereotypical and therefore less problematic.

## How to Enjoy Less Intensity

There's no doubt that the "better-half adventure" demands a certain degree of resignation to certain limitations. Self-image can change to allow for an appreciation of having more character in our faces. Hard-driving physical endeavors can give way to a more moderate approach to physical activity. Self-esteem can come from self-generated goals and accomplishments as opposed to grades, awards, promotions. Being recognized for competitive achievement can be replaced by the loving glow from the pleasure of seeing grandchildren or young relatives come into this world.

## The Contentment Factor

There's something very comfortable about the more relaxed approach to the "better-half adventure." We mellow out, as is often said. I call it the Contentment Factor—that commonly acknowledged loss of intensity as we ease into the comfort zone of life. There's some medical evidence to fortify this assumption: Between the ages of 40 and 60, scientists have found, there is a loss of cells in that part of the brain known as the *locus coeruleus*, a part of the brain which registers anxiety. What a pleasant gift nature has bestowed on us to make the "better-half adventure" more enjoyable!

# SIX YOUTH-EXTENDING ACTIVITIES

## 1. Call a Halt to the Madness

In the first half of life we are on a constant treadmill. According to a Harris survey, leisure time has shrunk, since 1973, a whopping 37 percent. During this same period, the average workweek has grown from 41 hours to 47 hours. The more ambitious professionals may end up putting in more than 80 hours per week, flitting from one stressful demand to another. Now, in the better half of your life, you can finally call a halt to such time-squeezing madness. You can relearn to enjoy life's leisurely pleasures—savoring the nuance of an old wine, enjoying the unrushed pleasure of a new-born relative, getting lost in a juicy, historical novel, or just plain ol' watching the sun actually set.

## 2. Enjoy the Harvest Years

The "better-half adventure" allows you the grace to return to the world what you gained in whatever good fortune you've had till now. Psychologists refer to this as the stage of *generativity*. You can now enjoy the continuous, ongoing process of life rather than perceiving it as a series of unrelated events. You can begin to connect with others because you care for them, not because you're forced to out of social or economic obligation. You can finally afford to live out the authentic values you always talked about in the abstract. You can now afford the time it takes to reconnect with your inner self, just by taking the space to relax and meditate.

During these "harvest years," you can bring together all your experiences to discover and express your special uniqueness to those you love and about whom you care. You've reached the prime of your spiritual life.

Accepting the concreteness of your mortality, you can savor each day for its precious opportunities for love and joy. Secure in the appreciation of your own values, you can now allow those different from you to be themselves without your having to judge them. You become more tolerant of differences.

## 3. Find the Meaning in Your Life

In midlife, you question the meaningfulness of your career, the occasionally felt emptiness in your life, and even the love in your marriage. Now you can reaffirm your close relationships, find your true calling as a vocation or hobby, and create the meaningfulness in your life you deserve.

Your search is for completeness. If you devoted the first half of life to career, you now have the freedom to find the nurturance of intimacy. If you chose to be a devoted, nurturing mother, you now have the freedom to unleash your drive to achieve a personal goal. If you wandered as an uncommitted, free spirit, you can now go back home or at least rebuild as much of it as you're able. Your quest is for wholeness, to bring back the missing part of your earlier half.

PERSONAL POWER BEGINS AT HOME. Personal power does begin at home, and extends outward, rather than the opposite. One of the most powerful of the Ten Commandments is to honor your parents, and by extension, your family. As you enter the "better-half adventure," you come home again in a spiritual sense. Whatever your early experience of family life, you can begin the process of forgiveness by posing the question: What is the source of your better qualities and your inner resources? The answer has to be your family of origin. Whatever fault you can lay blame on your family, it is also the source of your best and finest qualities.

## 4. Choose to Spend Time with Those You Admire

Once you've made peace with your family of origin, you're more capable of choosing and nurturing those relationships which truly nurture you back. Choose those you not only find attractive, but also whom you respect or admire; for it is with such individuals that you will find a shared value system and thereby the opportunities for greater personal growth. Choose to share time with these people. And if you live far apart, take to the fine old fashion of letter writing. Take the time to share what's in your heart. Such relationships, carefully nurtured, can grow over the years, enriching your lives in a mutual way.

## 5. Become Your Own Artist-in-residence

Allow yourself the luxury of becoming your own artist-in-residence. If you're musically inclined, buy yourself an instrument you've always liked and learn how to play it. Create your own music, to express the rhythms and melodies of your inner soul. If visual art is your choice, learn or relearn your favorite medium. At the very least, give yourself the opportunity to decorate your own living quarters with whatever appeals to the inner you.

## 6. Become an Author-in-residence

If you enjoy the written word, then you need no special instruments or equipment except for pen and pad, or if you're technologically inclined, a word processor or PC. You can write a newsletter pertaining to a particular passion of your own. You can write your soul-mate friends, giving yourself license to explore your inner self. At the very least, you can write to that most important individual: your very own self. We call it a diary or journal keeping. If you have a flair for the dramatic, try writing short stories about issues that pull at your heart strings. Or write a play. Enjoy the fantasy that a producer will get a hold of it, and beg you to allow him to make a film of it.

WRITE YOUR OWN STORY. I believe that everyone's life is a viable story in its own right. Explore your own issues, what makes you tick, what moral lesson is to be gleaned from your own life story. What really matters to you and what is to be done about it? If your life story points to some purpose, then this is the time for it to find expression, not tomorrow. Write your autobiography as if it were destined to be a best-seller.

Such self-expression and self-exploration can enhance the probability of living the full ten years longer and then some. According to Dr. Deepak Chopra, best-selling author of *Ageless Body, Timeless Mind*, six traits in particular are key for longevity:

1. Responding creatively to change.
2. Reducing anxiety.
3. Focusing on the ability to create and invent.
4. Maintaining high levels of adaptability and flexibility.
5. Integrating new things and ideas into your life.
6. Wanting to stay alive.

Finding a creative expression of your unique self affords you the opportunity to create and invent, integrate new ideas into your life, and respond creatively to change, especially if your creative outlet is writing.

In order to manifest your desire to stay alive, become more adaptable and flexible, and reduce anxiety, it's important to reduce stress in your life. This leads to our next section on staying younger by reducing stress within your family.

## HOW LOVE TURNS BACK THE CLOCK

Study after study reveals that having a close, supportive network reduces stress and promotes cardiovascular health. It's not only outside pressures that cause our blood pressure to rise; it's also the absence of supportive friends and family. Your closest relationships seem to matter most for your health. The more hostile you are during a marital argument, the harder it is on your immune system.

A study of stress using macaque monkeys came up with similar findings. The friendliest monkeys were found to have stronger immune responses while the most hostile and aggressive had the poorest. According to one of the researchers, "Affiliation protects animals from the potentially pathogenic influence of chronic stress."

### Have at Least One Friend from Whom You Hold Back Nothing

The number of supportive relationships is not as important as the quality of those relationships that do exist. In a nutshell, the lesson here seems to be: Nurture at least one or two highly supportive relationships in which you can totally be yourself, divulging your deepest secrets, holding back nothing. That's better than having fifty friends, and none with whom you can be completely open. And learn to be friendly, rather than hostile, cynical, and mistrustful.

### Learn How to "Fight Fair"

When couples fight for dominance, blood pressure rises. But when productive fighting occurs, for instance, to solve a problem rather than to gain dominance, blood pressure does not rise. Fair-fighting skills can help you avoid destroying your health. (See Chapter Four for eliminating the stress of conflict with your mate.) Struggles for dominance can lead to heart disease, but if your relationships are a source of comfort, they can exert a protective effect on your heart.

## DEVELOPING AN AGELESS OUTLOOK

You've heard that life begins at 40. In this book, you've realized how life can last ten years longer with a healthier lifestyle. You've also heard how youth is wasted on the young. Whether or not this is true, this chapter is about developing an ageless outlook during the mature years of your life—the part of your life that starts today.

As you mature, intellectually and emotionally, you can learn to be more assertive about your own needs. Having spent your early youth on a narrower perspective of humanity, you're now learning that a much deeper joy can be acquired by taking on a wider perspective of life. As you mature, it feels much better to be able to give to yourself as well as to others, supporting yourself emotionally, spiritually, and intellectually. You can be more prepared to take time to be aware of your deeper needs, to let them be nurtured and cared for, and to make use of the wisdom of your experience, continuing to feel ageless through the passing years.

This change in perspective as you mature out of the more formative years of your life not only nourishes others, it nurtures your own inner self in very significant ways. As you learn to reduce stress in your life through better communication with others, to be clear about your needs as well as being sensitive to those of your loved ones, you enhance your physical health as well. By reducing stress in your life you enhance your physical as well as mental health. As you acquire a more generous disposition toward your inner strength, you can look forward to a more meaningful and enjoyable longer life.

## SENSE OF PURPOSE

One of the key attributes of happy, long-living women is a sense of purpose in their lives. No matter what else transpires around them, these individuals do not lose their own sense of direction.

A sense of purpose can be described in both general and specific terms. At the general level, most people would agree on a common goal—to have our existence make a difference; to make use of the talents within us to make this earth a better place because of our being here; and to find deep meaning in our endeavors.

On a specific level, how that mission is carried out differs with each individual, and may change over time within each person. For many years, I felt my mission was to help others deal with their life challenges through the art and science of my profession. Now it appears my mission is being manifested in part through the written word. I write not only helpful books such as this, but dramatic pieces as well, both as a novelist and playwright. At this time of writing only one of my plays has been presented; but by the time you read these words, who knows?

As part of my education for writing drama, I recently took a course on writing screenplays. One evening, the instructor made a fascinating point about dramatic structure, which as I thought about it, also applied to real life. The protagonist or hero of any drama typically goes through a transformation to a "higher" level of being, and this transformation is not made by conscious decision. Rather, it is made—usually in the third act of a movie—when, just as the hero seems to be overcoming the challenge at hand, the worst of all possible outcomes happens. The rug is pulled out from under his or her feet, the world is turned upside down, making the previous challenge look like an anthill compared to the newly challenging Mt. Everest. Now the hero is ready for a *real* transformation.

If you recall the film, *Pretty Woman*, Julia Roberts plays the role of a prostitute who happens to come across a handsome financier, played by Richard Gere, who is lost in the byways of Hollywood. He pays her to help him find his way to his hotel. Almost as an afterthought, he invites her to be his social escort during his business stay.

Her challenge is to experience the transformation from common prostitute to sophisticated companion while, at the same time, allowing trust and love to break through the cynicism of her former lifestyle. Much of the film has to do with this early challenge. Just as she completes that flowering transformation what should occur but the most terrible possible outcome: She finds herself alone with her companion's lawyer, who attempts to force himself on her. When she resists he reminds her of her former status in hateful, crass terms, destroying her new-found pride and the blossoming love and trust. She decides to leave her companion despite the loving bond they've created. But the first transformation has already taken place. She returns home to pack her bags so she can leave her life of prostitution for more challenging options.

Having made this decision, what should occur but an opportunity for an even greater transformation. Her new-found-and-lost lover decides to make a critical detour in his own life and to offer her true, lasting love. Now it is she who must make a leap of faith and renewed trust. Her suitor asks what she will do now that he's come to save her and she answers "Save him right back"—realizing her final transformation from proud woman to healing woman. Her true sense of purpose has finally emerged.

## The Greatest Lesson—Discovering What We're All About

Think of your own life. Would you agree that only when the worst possible outcome challenges you, are you really forced to change? It is at such times that we are more open to discovering our inner purposes in life. The greater the challenge in life, the greater the lesson to be learned in finding out what we're really all about. It's the universe's way of getting our attention with a two-by-four upside the head and demanding: "Is this what your life is really all about? Wake up and look around!" We don't always make major changes through conscious decision—life forces us out of our ruts and demands that we look around for a more meaningful path.

## With Age, We Find More Learning Opportunities

As we get older, we find more learning opportunities—through dealing with failed relationships, professional setbacks, medical problems, and so on. Yet each cloud has its special silver lining, even thunderstorm clouds. As we mature, we're forced to explore our purposes.

## Joy Comes from Day-to-Day Relationships

As we mature emotionally, we may begin to realize that joy comes not from things, such as fast cars and wall-sized TV screens, but rather from the humble process of day-to-day relationships and how we choose to use our productive time. It's no longer the end result that matters as much, such as plaques on the wall or getting the better of someone, but rather the ongoing process of enjoying what relationships we do have and enjoying our work and play on a daily basis. Shakespeare says it so eloquently:

*"Things won are done, joy's soul lies in the doing."*
**—Troilus and Cressida, Act 1, Scene 2.**

## The More You Offer, the Less You're Hurt

The more open you are to exploring your deeper purpose in life, the less you will need undesirable outcomes to get your attention. The more you can embrace a sense of purpose, the less will you be susceptible. The most selfish individuals are those who are trying to hold on to control of their own lives and those of others—they are most susceptible to life's challenges. Those with a sense of purpose, generally to make available to others what they can offer, emotionally, spiritually, and intellectually, are least hurt by life's challenges. We can call this Ryback's First Inverse Law of Giving: The more you have to offer life, the less you're likely to be hurt by life. The same events may happen to the giver and the taker—illness, emotional loss, financial setback—but the giver is less hurt by such events.

## Givers Tend to Be Healthier, Less Greedy, and More Well-Liked

The giver's eyes are set on the purpose. As long as giving is still possible, whatever its medium, then life is still rich and meaningful, and illness, material loss, or personal insult takes on a relatively minor role. Paradoxically, however, those with a deep purpose of giving to others are more likely to remain healthy, free of material attachment, and well-liked by others. As we live a healthier, vital life for ten more years, it makes more sense to learn the deeper purposes of being a giver rather than a self-centered taker.

## Give to Others and You Will Feel Less Alone

Other than physical harm, the greatest source of stress is the sense of alienation we experience in life. A sense of purpose of giving to others removes that sense of alienation. As we give to others, whether it be through teaching, listening, or just being there for those who need us, we feel a connection with the life source and we become less susceptible to loneliness and rejection. We become less needy of material acquisitions and external symbols of achievement and more appreciative of the love and honesty we develop in our relationships and the comfortable sense of leisure that comes from enjoying whatever happens to be around us. We can enjoy our love for others, in its various forms and manifestations, as well as the challenge to discover those special qualities or talents unique to us as we choose to use them for the betterment of others, no matter how small that betterment may be. And, as Demosthenes points out:

> "No (wo)man can tell what the future may bring forth, and small opportunities are often the beginning of great enterprises."
>
> **—Ad Leptinem**

## Enjoying the Inner Self

The more we can rise above our petty desires and lift ourselves to the greater common good, the more we can trust our inner feelings to be true guides of our own behavior. Some call this intuition, others call it gut reaction. The more we free ourselves of petty desire and vulgar competition, the more sensitive we become to that inner guide that, over time, proves itself more accurate than intellect and logic. We become more comfortable with ourselves and enjoy time alone as a special treat rather than as loneliness. We may even choose to spend time with our inner selves in gardening, music, or meditation. Paradoxically, people seem to be more drawn to us now that we need them less. Ryback's Second Inverse Law of Solitude: The more you learn to enjoy your solitude, the more people are drawn to you.

## Giving Is Continual Fulfillment

There is so much we can attach ourselves to in terms of material objects or goals of achievement. We can never be satisfied if we continue to look away from ourselves, our own inner resources. External desire knows no end. A "house" as a symbol of success and achievement is never completed—it always needs more, to impress our neighbors. A "home" is accepted as it is—for its warmth and character, not to impress others. So it is with our lives. To impress others, we will never be completely satisfied. To have as our purpose to give to those around us, our lives are continual fulfillment. Harriet Sewall writes of this so beautifully, in her poem, *Why Thus Longing*:

> "Why thus longing, thus forever sighing
> For the far-off, unattain'd, and dim,
> While the beautiful all round thee lying
> Offers up its low, perpetual hymn?"

## You Can Be the Source of What Others Need

To live in need is to live in conflict—conflict between your desires and those of others—as if the world were running out of what you need. To live with purpose is to live as if you are the source of what others need. By choosing to live with purpose, you do indeed offer what others need. As you choose to live a longer, healthier life, you have the supreme gift of enjoying a "better-half adventure" and helping those around you to enjoy their lives as well.

## How to Achieve a Sense of Purpose

How can you achieve this sense of purpose? The answer is extremely simple. Just make claim to it! Take this very moment and make a claim to aspire to the purpose of offering yourself first to your loved ones—your mate, your children, and your parents—and start becoming aware of others' need for your love and acceptance. It's not your money or your cherished possessions or your time we're talking about, though they probably want at least some of those items.

## Don't Prevent Yourself from Showing Love

At a deeper level, they simply want to be accepted and appreciated by you. You probably do love and appreciate them, but are you preventing yourself from showing it? So the first step is to start with those closest to you.

Second, make peace with yourself. Learn to be more honest with yourself. Give up comparing yourself to others. Accept your shortcomings and allow yourself to become more appreciative of your uniqueness. There is no one exactly like you, never was, never will be, and this makes you uniquely special. Treat yourself to the experiences you really want, the music you like, the honesty you deserve with those you care about, the relationships with people you admire. Get to know your quieter self by spending quality time alone, in artistic pursuit, walking in nature, or just meditating in whatever way you most enjoy. By treating yourself as someone special, you'll begin to accept no less from others. You'll have less time for those who don't make you feel special. The quality of your life will grow in quantum leaps.

## LIVING MORE FULLY

Your fears will begin to dissipate, leaving you only with the inevitable fear of death and taxes. If you don't cheat on your taxes, that leaves you only with the fear of death. Here's Ryback's Third Inverse Law of Living Fully: The more fully you live your life, the less will you fear your death.

The more you put off for tomorrow, the greater your fear of losing tomorrow. The more life you enjoy today, the less you fear loss of the future. By living on purpose, you make each day, each moment, more real and significant. Tomorrow is more opportunity to give more to others. Your death becomes more their loss than your own.

### Empower Those Around You

As your mindset shifts from neediness to giving, your present life takes on more meaning and the future becomes an opportunity for more of your giving nature. In addition, you feel that your inner energies empower those around you. What you give away to others will live on beyond your physical demise. Although that sounds very philosophical, you can begin to get a sense of it and you can begin to feel a timelessness about your life.

So the "better-half adventure" of your life is directly ahead of you. It doesn't necessarily begin at 40; it can begin today, regardless of your age. One thing's for sure, there's no more time to be wasted. To the extent that you can learn to be more of a giver for those extra ten years, you'll have all the more to look forward to. Remember—the more you have to offer life, the less you're likely to be hurt; the more you enjoy your solitude, the more others want to be with you; the more fully you live, the less you have to fear. So enjoy yourself—the better half is yet to come!

## KEEPING YOUR MEMORY SHARP:
## FOUR QUICK TIPS

Enjoying your "better-half adventure" not only keeps your heart younger and healthier, it also keeps your mind active and healthy. The ability to remember, reason, and solve problems is superior in those over 60 who continue to exercise their faculties to the fullest.

As you age, neurologists say, part of your brain having to do with thinking and memory shrivels away at a rate of 10 percent per decade. Over a lifetime, the rate of transmission along neurons slows by about 10–20 percent. Yet, for those who stay fit, brain function can actually improve through middle age. How is this possible?

There are two reasons for this. The first is that the brain is full of redundant circuitry. There are many times the number of neurons we need to function at top level. So even though there is loss of brain process, there's more than enough left to pick up the slack.

The second reason is that the brain can be made to grow new neural connections through intellectual stimulation. Mental exercises can actually make the brain grow new nerve endings and more than make up for the losses due to aging. Use it or lose it, describes the situation well. Challenge your brain and you'll stay steps ahead of any loss due to aging. Here are four tips that will assure you a top-functioning brain.

### 1. Expect to Communicate Even Better as You Mature

According to neurosurgeon Vernon Mark, recently retired from Harvard Medical School, the mature person's brain can be prone to decline in certain complex areas of intelligence such as theoretical mathematics. However, intelligence in areas of applied skills does not decline, and certain areas such as art interpretation increase with time. Speech and writing abilities can actually improve through the 50s and 60s. Philosophers often don't hit their stride until age 70 or 80.

### 2. Add Mental Workouts to Your Physical Workouts

In addition to physical exercise, mental exercise also helps keep the brain in tip-top shape. To complement physical exercise for the body, consider the following mental workouts for top brain functioning.

Occasionally, balance your checkbook without the aid of a calculator. This will improve concentration and attention. If your mind is not otherwise occupied (during phone conversations, unimportant meetings), practice the fine art of creative doodling. Working playfully at geometric designs or simple cartoon-like drawings will improve perception of spatial relationships as well as enhance creativity. You might even graduate to the point of taking up drawing or painting, a wonderful creative expression that can be enjoyed into your 70s, 80s, and 90s.

## 3. A One-minute Memory Course

Memory can become problematic as you mature. One way of compensating for such loss is to combine a component of memory which does not decrease—music and verse—with the logical memory which does tend to decrease with age. By putting the items you want to remember in lyrics of songs you know very well, you can improve your memory beyond its original, younger state. Another technique, advocated by many memory experts, is to assign the numbers 1 through 7 to the various parts of your body (for example, 1 = head, 2 = eyes, 3 = mouth, 4 = chest, and so on.), and then associate items you would like to remember with those numbers and body parts. Silly associations are not only allowable, they're encouraged. If you have a grocery shopping list to remember, just imagine each item growing out of the assigned part of your body, and let yourself be silly about it. Imagine a loaf of bread growing out of the top of your head, having pears for eyes (a pair of pears), pearl onions for pearl white teeth, broccoli growing on your chest, and so forth. I'll leave the rest to your imagination.

## 4. Use of Acronyms—Roy G. Biv

Another memory technique is the use of *acronyms*, or taking the first letter of each item to produce a nonsense word which is easier to remember. You don't have to wait until you start losing your memory to age to begin acquiring this skill; a superior memory is desirable at any age. I can still remember the colors of the rainbow from the acronym "Roy G. Biv" I learned in elementary school—red, orange, yellow, green, blue, indigo, violet. Without Roy's help, I could never remember the definite order of the colors. From college, I remember the acronym OOTAFAGVSH for the spinal nerves without hesitation, though the individual nerves don't come back as readily. Optic, trigeminal, facial, glossopharyngeal,and vagus are all I can remember, not having thought of this for many, many years. Yet how amazing that I can recall that much after so many years in an instant, with the help of an acronym! The more you practice this, the more you'll have access to this lifelong skill. And so your memory will be just as good as ever, for the rest of your life.

## FOUR LIFE-EXTENDING QUALITIES

Such grace in the "better-half adventure," whether in making love or completing a personal project, does not fall gently upon us, but rather is a natural consequence of personal choice and determination. Left to our indolent and mindless habits of laziness, we can certainly expect the worst of aging with all its infirmity of body and vapidity of mind. But to take action against the evil ravages of old age is a powerful choice for extended youthfulness. Old age can certainly be a bitter and debilitating experience. Until our current generation, that's how it was typically considered. Certainly it has been thought of in this manner for centuries. Here's how Cicero considered it hundreds of years ago:

> As I give thought to the matter, I find four causes
> for the apparent misery of old age; first, it withdraws
> us from active accomplishments; second, it renders
> the body less powerful; third, it deprives us of almost
> all forms of enjoyment; fourth, it stands not far from death.

### Meeting the Challenge of the "Better-half Adventure"

Rather than a depressing dictum of dire decline, I see Cicero's comments as a challenge. If, during those special ten years, we can, first, stay active; second, remain powerful both in terms of body and mind; third, enjoy such powerful activity; and fourth, stay vital and engrossed in life rather than contemplate the inevitability of death, then the "misery" of "old age" can be transformed into the sweet experience of enjoying the "better-half adventure"— freer than ever to explore our talents to their fullest, to share our love without reservation with family and friends, and to push the edges of our vitality in whatever directions we choose.

## Stay Vital, Loving, and Engrossed in Challenge

Early in his career, the comedian Steve Martin once confronted his audience as it sat laughing uproariously at his zany humor: "Why are you all so happy? Don't you know you're all going to die someday?"

This sobering question only provoked more laughter, as well it should. Death is just as inevitable to the helpless infant as it is to the person of years. There's no advantage to hastening its approach nor to considering our demise too eagerly. By staying physically active, socially involved, and enjoying such activity to the fullest, no matter what our age, we defy Cicero's "apparent misery." We stay vital, happy, engrossed in the challenges and successes of life, maintaining our own health and energy through active choices, loving those closest to us openly and honestly, and supporting our friends and colleagues with the full use of the experience and wisdom of our years.

In celebrating his 75th birthday, General Douglas MacArthur shared with his audience the following description of youth, attributed to Samuel Ullman of Birmingham, Alabama:

> Youth is not a time of life—it is a state of mind. . . .
> It is a temper of the will; a quality of the imagination; a
> vigor of the emotions; it is a freshness of the deep springs
> of life. Youth means a temperamental predominance of
> courage over timidity, of the appetite for adventure over a
> life of ease. . . .

> Whether seventy or sixteen, there is in every being's
> heart a love of wonder; the sweet amazement at the stars
> and starlike things and thoughts; the undaunted challenge
> of events, the unfailing childlike appetite for what comes
> next, and the joy in the game of life.

So play well the game of life. Play it in your quest for fitness. Celebrate the food you eat with creative preparations. Respect the rules that govern the health of your body. Treat your playmates in life with similar respect. Love to the fullest, each day of your life!

# MINIMIZING
## LIFE PROBLEMS TO
## LIVE LONGER

## CHAPTER 12

Over and over, we hear and read about scientific evidence that reducing stress makes for a stronger immune system and a longer, healthier life. In order to live ten years longer, it's essential to reduce stress in as many areas of personal experience as possible. In this chapter you'll learn ways to overcome personal problems and to live a longer, happier life by dealing with life's challenges directly and forthrightly and to use your added years of maturity to support others in living longer, healthier lives with less stress as well.

## SEVEN SUGGESTIONS TO BUILD
## A STRONG SUPPORT NETWORK

This section is a review of some of the effective techniques mentioned earlier, brought together to form the basis of a rich, supportive personal network to be there through good times and bad. When problems do occur, you'll have friends to help you through them, so that stressful situations can be resolved quickly and effectively.

### 1. Be Helpful to Others so You Can Count on Them when You Need Help

Solid friendships are a two-way street. Only if both individuals are benefiting is the friendship strong enough to stand the test of time. The friendships you choose to foster can be maintained by ensuring that you offer at least as much as you get. For when you're in a pinch and needing your friend's help, it's unlikely that a promise to be a good friend from then on will do the trick. Only a history of mutual benefit will bear whatever strain your demands make at the time.

### 2. Have at Least One or Two Friends in Whom You Can Confide All Your Secrets Without Reservation

By now you know the importance of having at least one or two such friends. The freedom to unburden your soul when you're particularly troubled by matters you can't otherwise share freely, for whatever reason, is priceless. Again, such trust can only be built on a history of confidentiality shared between you.

For most people, confidentiality is a joke. Typically, the best way to spread news of unusual behaviors or circumstances is to tell it to someone and add, "but this is confidential," and then in a hushed tone, "super confidential." You can bet that the news will spread like wildfire, each person adding that urgent "super confidential" tag line that ensures the listener will rush to the next most intimate friend or lover and repeat the news, with slight distortion to add his or her own personal touch, again adding the tag line, "super confidential." It makes for a very efficient communication system.

The friends in whom you choose to confide are exceptions to this general rule. It may take years to build such trust and devotion, but the effort is well worthwhile. When the time comes, you'll have someone with whom to share your problems, and get a healthier perspective in all likelihood. In such fast friends, you have one of the most powerful of all stress-busters.

### 3. Don't Let Distance Be a Barrier—Use Letters, Fax, Phone, or E-mail to Communicate

One of the problems in nurturing such strong friendships is that you're not always lucky enough to have the good fortune of finding one in your immediate community. As your levels of responsibility and power grow, you're more and more likely to have opportunities for travel—to attend conventions, to meet clients, to offer seminars. You'll meet new friends and acquaintances and among these may be that special person you instinctively trust at some initial level. But he or she may live hundreds or even thousands of miles away. Usually that's enough to kill the possibility of a special friendship. But when it's not and you refuse to give up this opportunity, then you can easily overcome the distance between you by talking on the phone, sending faxes, or if you really want to be thoughtful with one another, good, old-fashioned letter writing. There's something about putting your feelings down on paper that's qualitatively different. It seems more personal and more permanent at one and the same time. So whatever form of communication you choose, you can easily overcome the distance between you and your special friend, especially if he or she is one of those special companions in whom you can open up without reservation, trusting implicitly in the bond of confidentiality between you.

### 4. Make It Your Business to Have Friends with the Expertise You May Occasionally Need

You alone are responsible for shaping the circle of friends you most desire. If you'd like this circle to be a resource of support to you in times of need, then the most direct way to assure this is to cultivate and foster such friendships. If you hesitate because of the fear that you might be using such relationships in a mercenary fashion, then think again about what I mentioned at the beginning of this section—any true friendship is based on mutual support. Think not what your friend can do for you, to paraphrase John Kennedy, think what you can do for your friend. Doctors, businesspeople, lawyers, and consultants need friends equally as much. What can you do for such friends? When you meet experts in fields of interest to you, and you genuinely like and trust these individuals, then reach out, ask some questions, and see if there's enough in common between you to invite friendship. And then think what you can do for your friend. It may be confidentiality, it may just be support offered during an occasional chat. But whatever it is, offer at least as much as you get.

## 5. Solve Your Problems on a Dependable, Routine Basis

Problems offer two options: one is worry, the other is solution. Many people procrastinate facing problems directly and choose to worry instead. That's a personal choice that you have in our free society.

The choice to solve your problems rather than go on worrying about them is made easier by the rich network of support you can now build. Choose one particular time of the week to work on solving your problems. My particular time is Friday mornings.

Whatever problems come up in my life, I relegate to work on them on Friday mornings, no matter what part of the week they may have arisen, barring fire and flood, of course, or similar crises that demand immediate attention. I set aside a few hours to size up the problem (I average about one or two a week) and decide on one of two possibilities: Can I solve the problem myself, or if not, whom can I contact who can either help me solve the problem directly or at least refer me to someone who can? I don't waste time burdening friends with my problems if they can't be of help in some way. (Of course, my special confidentiality friends hear of my problems any time we communicate, but these aren't the friends for Friday mornings, necessarily.)

In some cases, I may not call a friend at all, but rather an organization or agency that can provide me with special information. By waiting until Friday, I've had a chance to sleep on the problem, collect my thoughts (and anxieties sometimes) and focus sharply on constructive options.

## 6. Don't Waste Time on Individuals Who Drain You of Energy and Leave You Feeling the Worse for the Wear

Of course, everyone has a right to be unique, with all her special, individual characteristics. But some stand out as particularly draining. Occasionally, one such individual might be in a position to make demands for your attention even though you get annoyed and frustrated in this person's company. Even though you're adversely affected by this person, you might feel obligated to be available because of some special relationship, be it family, business, or merely because this individual happens to be a friend of a friend.

Without being overly rejecting, you can best handle such a dilemma by discerning exactly what this person wants from you. It may be just your blind attention to their ongoing rambling. If so, try to match this person up with another lonely individual with time on their hands so the two can form a satisfying relationship based on talking about whatever crosses their minds. Or this individual may be persevering about some personal problem to which they respond "Yes, but . . ." to each valuable suggestion with which you come up— annoying, after a while.

In this case, give this individual your best shot at whatever advice you consider most useful and then, if that advice is ignored, just excuse yourself by saying: "I've got to go now, but let me know when you've had a chance to follow up on my suggestions and we'll take it from there. But since I'll be fairly tied up for a while, please wait until after you've tried my suggestions before you get back to me."

In either case, you take responsibility for the value of your own time and you've done what you can to respond to your friend's needs. If you allow your time to be consumed fruitlessly on ways that frustrate and annoy you, then there's no one to blame but yourself. By being direct and as helpful as you can in a concise but constructive way, you enrich your friend all the more. And you free yourself up to spend your time more constructively, more enjoyably and, with less stress, to contribute to ten more healthy years.

## 7. Don't Resist Counseling or Psychotherapy When Any Problem Becomes Greater than You or Your Network Can Resolve

Occasionally, despite your concerted efforts and the support of your friends, a problem may arise that persists, causing you an unusual degree of anxiety. If, after a few weeks, such anxiety persists, consider talking to a psychotherapist. Such an individual is trained to listen attentively, consider all your lamentations, and help you reflect on your problem in such a way as to give you a liberating perspective.

In the end, the solution to your problem might be quite simple, but for some reason you've avoided it. That's probably why your friends' advice didn't help. You were blind to the obvious for some inner fear that you may have been harboring. A therapist's patient, sympathetic ear and calm, reassuring manner will help you face that inner fear and overcome it constructively. So when friends and your own personal resources occasionally fall short in solving a deep problem, don't resist a professional's help. This is a good fall-back position you can't afford to be without on at least some occasions in your life.

## PLAYING THE HAND THAT'S DEALT YOU

I hope I don't offend you with this, but it annoys me when I hear someone utter, after some unfortunate incident: "Well, things always work out for the best. There must be a reason for this (losing all one's money in an investment, having an expensive and painful accident, the death of a young friend) happening." It annoys me because such a statement preempts my feelings of anger or sadness. It also dismisses the meaning of the event by attributing an anonymous, meaningless "value" to it. If there is meaning to it, then let that be my own discovery, coming from my own consideration of thoughts and feelings. In other words, don't tell me there's a meaning to it before I've had a chance to acknowledge my own feelings and then let the personally felt meaning emerge naturally.

Don't dismiss personal failures out of hand by quickly saying: "Well, there must be a reason for that, but it's beyond me so I'll just go on with my life and pay no more mind to it."

Instead, find the opportunity for understanding, learning, and growth in each experience that may be initially painful and punishing. Whatever hand is dealt you, play it to the optimal. That means, whatever setback befalls you, play it back in your mind until you can discover the specific elements of your involvement that led to the unhappy results. This way, you grow by becoming more mindful and aware when in similar circumstances in the future. It's called wisdom.

Even negative emotions, apart from accidents and mishaps, can be transformed into positive feelings when the same mindfulness is applied. For example, consider envy, a negative emotion by anyone's standard. By exploring this emotion closely, you can transform it into a highly enjoyable one. Envy is a feeling of being deprived of something you notice in someone else's life. If you can change your perspective and encourage yourself to enjoy this other person's satisfaction in a vicarious way, then you'll be able to feel a modicum of joy instead of the pain of deprivation. By enjoying her success vicariously, you can ultimately share in that experience of success. Also, if your friend's success reminds you that you would like some of what he or she has, in addition to enjoying the success vicariously, find out (perhaps from him or her) what it takes, in terms of energy and focus, to acquire such success. You may even enlist your friend's support. Accept the hand that's dealt you, but if you choose a better hand, then you need to give up some cards from your own hand (time and energy), before you can pick up some unknown cards from the face-down deck (chance of success) to replace them. And whatever new cards you do pick up, play them as best you can, with confidence and optimism.

You determine your own success in many small, almost unnoticeable ways. Your life events can be predicted by your deeper expectations. Small and subtle behaviors accumulate to result in a decisive response, especially in social interactions. The more truly you expect something, the more your small and subtle expressions will result in the expected outcome. These small and subtle expressions communicate to others what's expected of them by you, and they typically oblige.

An obvious example of this is being stopped by a police officer for a traffic infraction. If you expect to be cited, the officer will happily oblige you. But if you truly feel innocent of the alleged infraction and your small and subtle expressions convey this, then the officer might just let you off with a warning. As a matter of fact, on a somewhat larger scale, that's what the legal jury system is all about. Six or twelve fellow citizens sit and watch the small and subtle expressions of the defendant and weigh these at least as heavily as the legal considerations of the case as they sort out their thoughts and feelings in the complex decision-making process. This is becoming more apparent as TV and print journalism analyze all the intricate components of the jury's decision-making process.

So by being increasingly aware of your true intentions and the subtle signals you convey to others, you can better play the hand that's dealt you. Go for what you want with what you have, directly and forthrightly. It's not a matter of luck. It's a matter of intention.

# SIX STEPS TO UNDERSTANDING OTHERS AT A DEEPER LEVEL

Richard, a highly intelligent, successful businessman in his early 40s, was having trouble in his marriage. Whenever his wife suggested something to him, he'd describe his own position in such abstract terms and with such earnest zeal that her idea became totally transformed in the process. A look of frustrated puzzlement would appear on her face and she'd withdraw emotionally for a day or two. She'd been through this so many times without any success of communicating with Richard that resignation was all she had left.

After a long talk with Richard, I convinced him that his style of communication might be great for persuasion at committee meetings, but that it was destroying his marriage. Poor Richard looked at me in amazement. But he was intelligent enough to pick up on my suggestions very quickly once he realized he needed to change at home.

Communication takes place at two levels—one level is the *face value* of the words spoken; the other is the *intent, motivation, fears,* and *desires* giving rise to the words expressed. By understanding the emotional origins of the words expressed, you're in the powerful position of cutting through such words to find their deeper meaning.

You can know this deeper level not by any trick or gimmick, but by the genuine effort put into understanding the other's perspective as much as possible.

But first you need to learn to be sensitive to your own motivation, fears, and desires so that you have a clear channel through which to recognize the feelings of others. This is not accomplished overnight, but by a continuing process of facing the truth of your own experience with brutal honesty. "To thine own self be true," and honesty with others will follow naturally. Then you can read others more clearly and openheartedly.

The next skill to be learned is to become articulate in expressing your own feelings with honesty and to help others feel safe and fulfilled through your incisive awareness of their deeper strengths and vulnerabilities.

To enter into the inner world of the person you want to understand more deeply, learn to put aside your own interests, at least temporarily. In this way, you can truly walk in another's shoes.

The word "understand" can be broken down into the words "standing under"—seeing the world from the other's unique, personal perspective. Only by forsaking your own perspective for the moment can you truly understand the other. Most people are unable to accomplish this. You can, if you devote yourself to the process. Here's how.

1. In your conversation, repeat what you've heard as if you had become the other. Pretend in your own mind that the other person has temporarily lost his or her ability to speak and you're doing your best to speak for him or her. Repeat what you've just heard as accurately as possible, repeating the exact words if possible, or paraphrasing as closely as you can. You can start off saying, "If I hear you right, you're saying that . . . ."

2. Having done this to the best of your ability, now check to see if there's accuracy in your perception. "Is that right?" or "Am I on target?" or "Do I understand what you're saying?"

3. You may be surprised to discover that you're off target a lot more than you expected, especially when you first start out. People think they hear more accurately than they typically do. Keep repeating steps 1 and 2 until you do get a response that tells you you're close to being on target. Now you're ready for step number 3: Report the feeling or emotion you feel lies behind the other's statement, for example, "It feels as if you're angry (sad, hurt, ecstatic, etc.) about this," and follow up again with a check for accuracy, "Is that right?"

4. Always go with the other's corrections and forget about being right or wrong.

5. This is not about winning a debate—it's about getting close to the other so you can better understand him or her. As you continue in that process, be as openly supportive as you can in both manner and tone of voice. Maintain good eye contact and lean gently toward the other, with attentive interest. Avoid mak-

ing any judgments about what you hear. Pretend you're inside the skin of the other, seeing things exactly the way he or she does.

6.  Don't fear losing your own self, even though you're letting go of your own values and judgments temporarily. Your value system will still be there after the conversation, and you'll actually become emotionally stronger in the process, with a somewhat more flexible, enlightened outlook on life. Having entered the perspective of another, your own perspective is now broadened.

As I continued my talks with Richard, he learned to use his quick mind to adopt this new, exciting form of communication with his wife. "I realize I've been in my own head all this time," he admitted. "I just never stopped to think about it this way before." After a while, Richard was using this new style of communication to overcome some problem relationships at work that had resisted his otherwise successful business style. Now Richard's marriage was like a second honeymoon and he was gaining a new kind of respect at work as well. His success both at home and at work was no longer hampered by his former inability to read other people.

As you foster this skill of understanding others better, including your mate, children, boss, and co-workers, you'll have considerably less stress in your life and you'll be adding another component to a longer, healthier life, not to mention greater happiness personally and more success professionally.

## GOING WITH THE FLOW

Just as you can be sensitive to another's thoughts and feelings, so can you be sensitive to the changing and challenging events in your life. By giving up a rigid view of life and being open to the varied possibilities and their potential benefits, you can more easily adapt yourself to whatever challenges confront you.

Consider that there is no absolute truth. Certainly there are laws that, when broken and enforced, result in punishment. But at a more personal and philosophical level, the deepest truths are not easily captured in fixed rules. If there is one rule that leads to true happiness, it has more to do with genuineness and honesty than any other style or quality.

Any decision that can go either way, for instance a dilemma, usually has no inherent correct answer. Either way is probably okay. By investing your ego in one way, you may lose. By accepting either outcome as equally viable, you free yourself from attachment. Instead of deciding with your head, allow your heart to be open to both outcomes. Accept the one that emerges naturally as you support the welfare of others rather than your own selfish attachments.

A short time ago, I was to give a reading from a novel I'd written. The reading was to take place in a large auditorium. Concerned that so few people would attend that the audience would feel dwarfed by the large auditorium, a smaller room was reserved as an alternative. The day before the reading, however, a decision had to be made because of the time restrictions in setting up video cameras and lighting. I wanted the more professional lighting available only in the auditorium, so that the video would have a more professional look. On the other hand, the audience would, in all likelihood, feel more comfortable in the smaller room.

Overlooking my own selfish concerns, I intuitively chose the smaller room. When the time for the reading finally came, it became quite apparent I'd made the "right" choice, even taking my selfish concerns into consideration. What happened was that a technician-in-training had been assigned to run the camera. When my reading finally began, the individual in charge of the evening witnessed a painful look on the technician's face. Without hesitation, she rushed up to the technician to realize that she couldn't find the button that would start the recording. A couple of frantic phone calls later, the problem was resolved.

When I discovered this at the end of my reading, after a few moments of anger and disappointment, I realized that the problem could be resolved by recording the first ten minutes of the reading (the part originally missed) over again, even though the audience had already gone. This was simple enough to do. After editing, the end result might even be better.

Now, had I chosen the more selfish alternative to read in the larger, but darker auditorium, the person in charge would never have been able to see the look of desperation on the face of the shy technician. The whole reading would have transpired without the correct record button ever having been found. And my hoped-for tape would never have been made. Moral? When faced with a dilemma, you never really know which choice is the better. If the pull to either side is about the same, choose the one that benefits others as well as yourself. Chances are it'll come out better for you as well.

---

# RISING ABOVE THE FURY: FOUR STEPS TO CONQUERING STRESS AND ANXIETY DUE TO MAJOR CRISES

---

Despite the best of intentions and the most open of hearts, occasionally life deals a devastating blow. Whatever the nature of the threat, or loss, the adrenaline flows, sleep is lost, and anxiety pervades. What to do to cope with such threats?

1. Imagine the worst possible outcome and the consequences of that. If that worst outcome is death, then you can surrender yourself to the profession and technology of medicine and accept such support. If the outcome is financial ruin, then consider how you would accept a different level of material consumption. If the outcome is legal prosecution, then consider how justice prevails, and accept your punishment or assert your innocence. In most cases by far, the outcome is not so severe, but by considering the worst, you can more easily deal with the rest.

2. Solicit the support of the most capable professionals available to you—doctors, lawyers, financial experts. Follow their expertise.

3. Realize the ultimate rule of overwhelming problems: This too shall pass. At least you have a chance. You can't lose anything by banking on that chance.

4. Having done all this, accept the anxiety as just another experience of life. And watch it disappear.

## HEALTHY PROBLEM SOLVING

In Chapter Three, I focused on how to initiate and maintain an effective fitness program.

One factor outweighs all others in acquiring and maintaining a healthy body—a desire to participate in and enjoy disciplined physical activity that is challenging and satisfying. The key is to enjoy such activity and to experience a sense of fulfillment as one goes from level to level of challenge.

A fit and healthy body makes all challenges somewhat more approachable. With more vigor and energy, intellectual, administrative, and creative efforts are tackled more easily. In addition, being fit contributes to a greater sense of self-esteem.

A moderate, ongoing involvement in an enjoyable activity can be little effort, once the routine is well-established. For those women who enjoy challenge or competition, fitness activities such as team sports and footraces provide these. A brisk walk is excellent for those who don't take to intense activity.

The key is to develop an appetite for physical activity, if it isn't yet developed. Once fitness becomes part of your life, and you experience the stamina, energy, and confidence that result, you're a step ahead in terms of solving your personal problems.

## SHARPENING YOUR INTUITION TO HELP YOU MAKE BETTER DECISIONS

To begin with, intuition and gut feelings are typically more reliable and trustworthy in the long run than what your brain can tell you. Your brain works with all the data you're aware of. Your intuition includes all these data and then some, such as data you have in your brain, but that you can't articulate in thoughts or words. These subconscious data are at the feeling level.

You can't remember everything you see and hear, but all data that enter your brain through your senses are virtually trapped there till you die. You can only put into words or conceptualize a tiny fraction of all the data trapped within your skull. The part that you can put into words is what psychologists refer to as *conscious mind*. All the rest—the data that can't be expressed in words because they haven't been processed by certain components of the "thinking" cerebral cortex—is called the *unconscious mind*.

When you decide with your thoughts alone, you're using only a small fraction of all your brain data. When you use your intuition to help you decide, you're able to use more data that you can't put into words, yet you can still sense through your bodily feelings. This is what women refer to as "intuition" and what men call a "gut feeling." Since intuition uses bodily feelings as well as conceptual data, more data is available, therefore resulting in a better or "smarter" judgment or decision.

In order to foster such intuition and "inner wisdom," begin by taking some time each day to meditate in a comfortable setting, free from distraction, and free from any attempts at problem solving. In this way, you can begin to tune in to all the data that are not otherwise available and feed them into the decision-making process. You can then expect to make sounder decisions and wiser judgments.

## MINIMIZING PERSONAL CONFLICT BY EXPRESSING GRATITUDE

Expressing gratitude is a simple yet very effective habit for making all your relationships run much more smoothly. In this way, you can strengthen the sources of support that enrich your life. You can consolidate that positive stream of giving that makes you feel more secure and fulfilled. Start with those closest to you. The closer the relationship, the more warmly expressed the gratitude.

There are many overlooked possibilities for expressing gratitude within your own family. When your mate helps you with the dishes, office work, or other chores, does he feel taken for granted? He won't if you make a habit of thanking him. What about your children? Do you think they'd be more likely to clean up their rooms or take out the garbage if you remembered to thank them on a consistent basis? Personal conflicts within your family might be reduced considerably by such simple measures.

It is similar with co-workers. If you remember to thank them for the little acts of assistance and consideration that come your way, then these helpful acts will only increase and endure. Thanking your subordinates for fulfilling their duties is nothing less than good management.

What about gratitude expressed to your superiors? Sound odd? An occasional brief note, sincerely expressed and sincerely felt, expressing appreciation for a policy decision you truly support, can let them know that you're comfortable being a team player. Of course, if you're at all oversolicitous in your tone, this can come across as brown-nosing. But if you can express your gratitude concisely and with a professional tone, then such communications can only do you good.

If your life is going fairly well, and you do appreciate that it is, a general attitude of gratitude can be expressed by small and large acts of generosity to those not yet in your support network—to life as a whole. This expression can emanate toward those you serve in your job or career. This attitude can only enhance your relationships with those you serve and make your life work more meaningful and enjoyable.

Reducing interpersonal conflict comes from your attitudes and actions, by performing deeds and saying things that contribute to richer, more meaningful relationships, to a greater sense of self-esteem and ultimately to a fulfilling sense of purpose or mission.

The more you can acquire the habit of expressing gratitude, through appreciating and supporting others, the happier you'll feel, and the healthier your mental state and physical well-being.

## BECOMING A BETTER PROBLEM SOLVER BY BECOMING A VOLUNTEER

As an extension to acquiring the habit of expressing gratitude, you have the opportunity to contribute aspects of your energy and talents to organizations, be they health-care agencies, professional organizations, educational institutions, or political parties. You can volunteer to help the sick or needy, support the organizations that represent your job or profession, teach or coach some inner talent you enjoy sharing, or support the candidacy of politicians who express your values.

Despite my busy lifestyle, I'm committed to offering my services as a voluntary contribution to at least one or more organizations. In the past, I've been a speaker for the American Cancer Society, a national cancer organization, and other health-oriented societies. I've done counseling at a local church, as well. More recently, I've donated my time as an organizational consultant to the government of the county in which I live. This activity has not only given me the opportunity to meet a number of interesting and effective administrators, but also put me in touch with sources of support which I might need at some time in my life. Beyond that, I enjoy a sense of civic pride, knowing that I can be a helpful part of my local government. You can do this too, without waiting to be appointed or going through a campaign for election. Just offer the best of what talents you have and the skills you've acquired. There's always room for a good and effective volunteer.

Here is how becoming a volunteer will both help you become a better problem solver and help minimize personal problems:

1. You'll have the opportunity to meet interesting, influential and typically supportive individuals who can be models for you to become a better problem solver. These typically successful individuals can also be models for dealing with life's problems by avoiding them through foresight and appropriate preventive measures.

2. You'll have an opportunity to explore your hidden potential— resources and talents heretofore undeveloped. The demands made on you may be very different than those with which you're familiar in your regular work, releasing a side of you that would otherwise remain untapped.

3. You'll gain more experience in assuming responsibilities that are new to you and in coordinating your talents with those of others. Such new talents and coordinating skills will definitely make you more efficient at solving problems and paving the way for smooth personal relationships.

4. By interacting with people with diverse lifestyles and different perspectives, you'll broaden your own perspective and become more understanding of other points of view. This broader perspective will make you a better problem solver and minimize conflicts due to differing viewpoints.

This habit of contributing to social, professional and political organizations should be fostered until it becomes strongly ingrained. As personal problems and interpersonal conflict become more easily resolved, you'll feel happier and more fulfilled.

By following the suggestions and examples I've offered in this chapter, you can not only get rid of personal problems as they occur and prevent many from occurring in the first place; you can also look forward to living a life of dignity and fulfillment, enjoying richer and deeper relationships with those at home and at work—a life of the highest quality, given your circumstances. Appreciate the uniqueness of every individual you come across; stay in touch with special friends, no matter where they live; listen with your heart as well as your head; and know when to lean on others. When your cup fills to the brim, give some back in terms of appreciation, gratitude, and some form of service to your community. You'll get it back, in spades. And a life of more joy and less stress will help you live ten years longer as well.

---

I've done my best to provide you with the most useful and practical information to help keep you living ten years longer and looking ten years younger. But additional information keeps coming up as research continues on this most vital subject. In order for you to stay abreast of the latest news and information on this topic, I've initiated a monthly information update to keep you at the cutting edge with the least effort on your part. A free sample of the *Live Longer Newsletter* is available at the following address:

Dr. David Ryback
1534 N. Decatur Road
Atlanta, Georgia 30307

I hope to hear from you.

# INDEX

# C̲

# O

Oats, 35
Obesity:
  and heart disease, 244
  and reproductive system cancer, 180
Oily skin, cleansers for, 213
Omega-3 fatty acids, 202, 255
One-minute memory course, 305
Onions, and arthritis, 202
On-the-job stress, 102-4
Oophorectomy, 145-47
  good reasons for having, 146
  and osteoporosis, 186
  recuperating from, 147
Optimism, developing, 15-17
Oral administration, estrogen, 139
Orgasms:
  and exercise, 73-74
  faked, 157
  multiple, 156
  simultaneous, 155
  without erection, 157
Ornish, Dean, 253, 264
Osteoarthritis, 200
  supplementation for, 203
Osteoporosis, 128, 140, 183-94
  and bone remodeling process, 184-85
  and calcium, 188-90
  definition of, 183-84
  Dr. Ryback's Osteoporosis
    Prevention Diet, 189, 201
  and exercise, 186, 190-94
    aerobic activities, 192
    non-aerobic activities, 192
    stretching, 192-94
    weight lifting, 194
  Osteoporosis Sensitivity Test, 187-88
  risk factors for, 185-87
Osteoporosis Sensitivity Test, 187-88
Ovarian cancer, 180-81
Ovaries, and estrogen production, 126
Overhead press, 194
Ovulation, 126

# P

PABA, 68
Painful intercourse, 131
Palm oil, 252
Pantothenic acid, 68
  and arthritis, 202
Pap smear, 179
Parathyroids, 185
Parkinson's disease, 50
Parlodel, 175
Partner:
  finding, 15
  for quitting smoking, 280
Pasta, 35, 52-53
Pauling, Linus, 41-42
Peanut butter, 32
Pears, 55
Peas, 53
Penicillamines, and arthritis, 201
Pergonal, 175
Perimenopause, 125
Personal conflict, gratitude expressed
  to avoid, 322
Personal power, 293
Pesticides, 55-56
  and pregnant women, 65
Petroleum jelly, as a moisturizer, 219
Phosphorus, 48
pH scale, 218
Phytochemicals, 29
Piracetam, 50-51
Placebo effect, 288-89
Pollutants, and pregnant women, 65
Polyunsaturated fats, 53, 252-53
Poor nutritional habits, converting,
  24-25
Popcorn, 32, 35, 53, 55
Porcelain veneers, 237
Post-menopause, 125
Potassium, 48, 69, 180, 258-59
Potato chips, substitutes for, 32
Power breakfasts, 27
Power foods, 38-40
  beta-carotene in fruits and
    vegetables, 39-40